Healthy Fitness Central

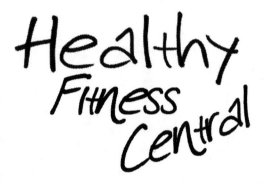

The Essential Guide for Fitness Training wherever you are! Home Workouts, Training at the Gym, Track or Swimming Pool, from Fitness Guru Christin McDowell

By Christin H McDowell

Visit us on the web at:

www.HealthyFitnessCentral.com
www.ChristinMcdowell.com
www.TrishaStewart.com

ISBN 978-0-9816846-2-8

Books by Trisha Stewart include:

      Healthy Tart
      Healthy Dude Book
      Healthy Idol
      Healthy Bunch Cookbook

Dedication

This book is dedicated to the people out there who can't live without exercise and are as crazy about working out as I am!

Acknowledgements

Special thanks to Christine Ely and the whole Waterleaf Publications team, Dr. Tim Burnham, Dr. Harry Papadopoulos and all the Central Washington University Exercise Science Staff.

Contents

Introduction	8
Chapter 1 - The PROCESS of REAL Weight Loss	10
Chapter 2 – Assessment	12
Chapter 3 - Men's Fitness	23
Testosterone	27
Training	29
- Overweight Men	32
- Average Joe	41
- Super Jock	48
- Skinny Beans	52
Chapter 4 - Women's Fitness	56
Severely overweight	63
Android Women	67
Gynoid Women	76
Chapter 5 - Stability and Balance Training	87
Chapter 6 – Stretching	101
Chapter 7 - Pregnancy and Fitness	109
Chapter 8 - Myths, Q & A	113
Chapter 9 - Exercise Equipment	117
- Track Workouts	120
- Pool Workouts	123

Contents (continued)

- Exercise Reference Section   127

     Back   (Exercises for)   127

     Bosu Ball   136

     Biceps   142

     Chest   146

     Core   159

     Jack Your Heart Rate   171

     Legs   175

     Medball   195

     Physioball   199

     Shoulders   206

     Track   214

     Triceps   223

Afterword   227

Healthy Fitness Central

Introduction

> *"Lack of activity destroys the good condition of every human being, while movement and methodical physical exercise save it and preserve it."* Plato

You've made it this far. You've decided to get more information on working out! For some of you, your fitness crusades may have involved purchasing precarious devices that promised weight loss and toned abs, but have gotten you nowhere except for some damaged nerves!

So you smartened up and decided to put some actual work in; you crunched your little abs 'til they could crunch no more... To your surprise and dismay, your belly is as big as it ever was, and actually, seems a bit bigger!

Chances are you spent a fortune joining a gym (or buying your own home gym), but ended up frustrated and de-motivated as you did nothing with it; just like thousands of others! So unless something happens soon, like now, you'll turn to the dark side and accept defeat; or worse, spend thousands of dollars stapling your stomach or sucking your fat out. Whoa! Bad choice! But that's not you is it?

Congratulations. The fact that you're reading this book means that you've made the right choice to *change your body for life*! So breathe a sigh of relief. I will show you from start to finish, what you need to do to progress your body from where it is right now, to the strong, healthy and vital body you yearn for!

Healthy Fitness Central is a book that works for everyone. I have specific sections devoted to men and to women as well as particular body types and special needs. Attaining a level of personal fitness is far more important than just looking good.

Being fit will enhance the quality of your life as well as extending it. I have a tag line for my fitness company which is 'Change your body for life!' I want you to have a better quality of life through good nutrition, a healthy lifestyle and plenty of the right kind of exercise. I want you to look good and to live long!

This book will help you achieve your goals of losing weight, gaining muscle mass and improving your general lifestyle. It will enable you to achieve fitness levels that you always have hoped for, but may not have thought possible.

Healthy Fitness Central

Healthy Fitness Central provides a structured program to help you achieve your goals regardless of your current state of fitness. I take my clients' and readers' health very seriously which is why I spent years studying to gain the necessary qualifications and experience to provide the best level of training possible. I have a degree in exercise science; I'm a certified strength and conditioning specialist and over the years have trained many people of different body types.

My background is in sports performance science which I have carried into my personal training techniques. I feel such movement patterns and mechanics can and should be universally practiced. Don't worry if you're not an athlete, this book will work for you! It has everything you need to know about attaining real fitness.

Get ready! You're are about to be handed the keys that can change your body and quality of life forever!

Why I chose to write this book

I see too many people eating too much junk food, drinking too much carbonated sugar water, spending too much time sitting on their ever expanding behinds, only to collapse on the sofa at night with a pizza and a beer to watch the latest episode of 'The Biggest Loser'. Face it America; we're gettin' fatter and we're suffering because of it!

Our kids are getting diabetes, liver transplants and premature puberty for Pete's sake, and we're not doing any better ourselves! Studies show that by 2015, 75% of the adult population will be overweight and nearly half of those will be considered clinically obese.

People are dying from their over indulgent and sedentary life styles, but it doesn't have to be like this!

Healthy Fitness Central can be used as a standalone fitness training tool, but is also part of the 'Healthy Lifestyle' series of books brought to you by Waterleaf Publications. The information contained in these books provides you with EVERYTHING needed to achieve a sustainable healthy lifestyle; for you and your family.

Chapter 1

The PROCESS of REAL Weight Loss

There's no easy way out. If there were, I would have bought it. And believe me, it would be one of my favorite things!" Oprah Winfrey

Here we go!

Do you know how many internet sites, books, magazines and advertisements I could cite that claim you can lose 20lbs of fat in a week? Too many... so let me make this clear; the only thing you are losing is muscle, water, poop, pee, nutrients, minerals, vitamins and oh, the money it took to try the quick fix. Real weight loss requires <u>real work</u> with real changes. Each pound lost takes time, physical work and/or restraint.

When you move you burn calories, which in the end, provided you don't eat it all back, means you will lose fat and keep it off. Weight loss takes physical WORK, and that my friends, is what you need to do!

Thankfully, my friend and colleague Trisha Stewart has provided all you need to know about proper nutrition in her books Healthy Tart, Healthy Idol and the Healthy Dude Book. Also, check out her website at www.trishastewart.com, a huge resource for all your nutrition requirements.

Fitness is far more than just burning calories. Being fit improves every functioning aspect of your body: your organs, muscles, digestive system, brain, bones, emotions, memory, alertness, sleep patterns and much more!

Fitness is not doing the same boring exercise day after day but rather involves progression, variety and performing things your body was made to do! Examples would be running, swimming, hiking, skiing, climbing etc! Because it's my goal to make you lose weight and become FIT at the same time, I have provided a comprehensive and progressive set of workouts made for all body types, ages, and levels of fitness.

Many of you will already know the benefits of cardiovascular work and weight training... however you need to know why it's good for YOU; specifically for your body type and gender. The chapters and articles in this book address all of your unique workout needs and for clarity are divided into sections of men's fitness and women's fitness.

The Men's Fitness sections have workouts for all types and sizes of men which include:

- The obese
- Moderately overweight
- The Average Joe-who by the way is basically overweight
- The Super Jock

It doesn't matter which one you are, as there will be workouts and explanations for your particular needs. Super Jock can't train the same way an Obese Man can, and an Obese Man should NOT train like Super Jock; maybe down the road, but definitely not now.

Women's Fitness sections cater for 2 types of Women:

1. 'Androidian' Apple (Belly) Fat Woman!
2. 'Gynoider' Pear (Butt and Thighs) Fat Woman!

Ladies, you MUST train for your body type. You will respond differently than men and from each other. Therefore, your workouts MUST be specific for your body type and level of fitness. There are timelines, programs, recommendations and explanations that assist you in your journey toward fitness.

Getting Started:

You need to start off with some simple steps by:

1. Figuring out your Heart Rate Prescription
2. Doing a Muscular Imbalance Assessment and learn how to "Retract"
3. Getting the proper shoes and inserts if you need them!

The next chapter will discuss what these are, why they are important and how to do them. Then you'll find yourself jumping right in to the specifics of making yourself fit for LIFE!

Chapter 2

Assessment

Target Heart Rate Zone, Heart Rate Reserve

The following is an illustration that I want you to look at and assess yourself with. The purpose of this illustration is to give you a BASE Target Heart Rate Zone or Heart Rate Reserve. What the heck? You've probably heard of Heart Rate Zone, but what the heck is Heart Rate Reserve? Well, I am glad you asked!

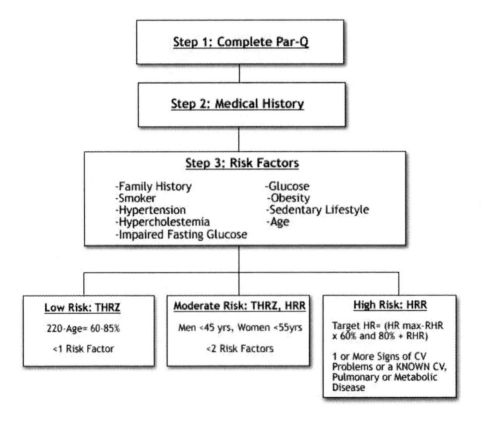

Health Screening and Heart Prescription

(HR prescription will depend on Health History)

Step 1: Complete Par-Q

Step 2: Medical History

Step 3: Risk Factors

-Family History
-Smoker
-Hypertension
-Hypercholestemia
-Impaired Fasting Glucose

-Glucose
-Obesity
-Sedentary Lifestyle
-Age

Low Risk: THRZ

220-Age= 60-85%

<1 Risk Factor

Moderate Risk: THRZ, HRR

Men <45 yrs, Women <55yrs

<2 Risk Factors

High Risk: HRR

Target HR= (HR max-RHR x 60% and 80% + RHR)

1 or More Signs of CV Problems or a KNOWN CV, Pulmonary or Metabolic Disease

Before starting an exercise program, you should always double check with your doctor to make sure you're healthy enough to start a fitness training program, no matter the difficulty. He or she will do a full evaluation to make sure everything is right and working.

The next step is to use this illustration, which shows whether you should use the Heart Rate Reserve (HRR) Formula or Target Heart Rate Zone (THRZ) as the base line for your heart rate.

If you have been sedentary for the greater portion of your life, or if you have any kind of existing condition such as high blood pressure, diabetes, etc., it is very important to monitor your heart rate for the first 3-6+ months of 'working out'. When you start out, don't work too hard.

The next thing is Risk Factors. Count how many things you have in the Risk Factor box (which is shown on the illustration) and assess if you are at Low, Moderate or High Risk.

- Low Risk: THRZ (60-85%)
- Moderate Risk: THRZ, HRR (60-78% THRZ), (60-80% HRR)
- High Risk: HRR (60-80%)

Classify yourself!

THRZ: TARGET HEART RATE ZONE

What is it? THRZ is a formula designed to give people a heart rate range (in beats per minute) during exercise. It is for individuals who have been cleared to exercise with no heart problems or risk factors. (See Illustration below).

So this **excludes** people with:

- high blood pressure
- known heart problems
- a sedentary lifestyle
- obesity
- and any known Risk Factor

What is my THRZ?

Well it's pretty easy to figure it out.

220-(Your Age) = 54 x .6 = Low HR beats/min

220-(Your Age) = 54 x .85 = High HR beats/min

Example: 35 year old Healthy Tart

220-35= 185 x .6= 111

185 x .85=157

So your range is (111-157) beats/min!

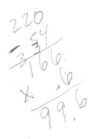

Fact/Fiction:

So you know how almost all of the elliptical/cross trainer exercise machines these days have THRZ monitors on them, and refer to the "Fat Burning Zone" and the "Cardiovascular Zone"? Throw that out! Losing fat is all about burning calories. You do the math! At a lower HR, sure you are burning more calories from fat, but you aren't burning that many.   At a higher HR, you're burning more TOTAL calories, you're improving your body's ability to use fat as its primary energy source and you're improving your cell's ability to sustain and transport oxygen more efficiently (which will lower your RHR and blood pressure).

Chances are that in your 'Fat Burning Zone' you're not even breaking a sweat, at least I'm not. So feel free to step up the intensity when you're ready. You can potentially reach a THRZ of 220-AGE!

Of course I am not recommending that right away, but a sign of superior physical fitness is to be able to reach that mark safely. Start off slow and progress comfortably, but remember that you can improve.

Recommendation:

- Train at least 3x/wk for 45min. to live longer
- To lose body fat, the accepted recommendation is to train 5-7x/wk for 60min.

HRR: Heart Rate Reserve

It's a Heart Rate formula, just like THRZ, but is typically used for people who have had any complications with their health.

The differences between the THRZ and this method is HRR takes into account YOUR resting heart rate AND your age.

Who uses this formula?

Again, it is generally used for people who have had health problems like: high blood pressure, heart problems, sedentary lifestyle etc.

What is my HRR?

Target HR = (HR max – RHR) x.60 and .80 + RHR

(HR Max is 220-age)

*Adjust the percentages of intensity depending on your RHR, medical history, current level of fitness, and the consistency of your past workouts. If your history is really poor, lower the percentages, (e.g. 50%-70%).

Remember that both of these prescriptions are GUIDELINES

If you experiencing shortness of breath, feel like your HR range is too hard, or too easy, adjust your heart rate level immediately. I would also ask your doctor if he or she thinks your HR range is adequate for you. Also visit www.trishastewart.com to ask me any questions.

If you have shortness of breath within your prescribed HRR or THRZ, feel you are getting dizzy or clammy, please adjust your workout. Slow down, stop, or take a break. It is EXTREMELY important to your well being and longevity that you progress within a safe manner. The WORST thing you can do is start off too hard. If you have had a history of high blood pressure and heart issues, as I said before, START OFF SLOW. Allow your body to adjust to this new stimulus. It is much better to have a lower heart rate and go longer than to have a higher heart rate and push your system too hard.

Muscular Imbalances!

A muscular imbalance is exactly what it says it is: an imbalance of muscular strength. It is where the muscle has not been adequately strengthened or is working too much, which will result in abnormalities of posture or body mechanics. Muscular imbalances can be corrected by stretching certain muscles and strengthening weak targeted muscles.

How do I know if I have one?

If you have a muscular imbalance you are much more likely to experience some of the following problems:

- Lower Back Pain
- Specific Hip Pain/Tightness
- Knee Pain
- Neck Pain/Tightness
- Chronic Injuries
- Limited range of motion when stretching

Typically you will notice that you are always tight in a certain area. You may experience excessive soreness, chronic injuries, limited range of motion when stretching, or extreme pain. The most blatant problem that screams "muscular imbalance!" to me is multiple knee surgeries.

Sometimes you'll have such a long history of being tight in a certain region; you just forget about it, so doing the assessments is a great way to see if there is something going on.

LARGE NOTICABLE MUSCULAR IMBALANCES:

1. Protracted Shoulder girdle: Your shoulders slump forward
2. Anterior Pelvic tilt: "Swayback", Your butt sticks out and your lower back seems to cave in towards your stomach
3. External rotation of foot: You walk with your feet coming out, like a duck
4. Knee Knock: Your knees knock together when you sit down, jump or squat
5. Forward Head tilt: Your neck sticks forward
6. Ankle/Ankles fall inward

ASSESSMENT:

1. Overhead Squat
2. Watch the way you walk
3. Look at the way you stand

BASIC QUESTIONNAIRE:

1. Do my feet turn out when I walk?
2. Do I look like I am always slouching?
3. Are my hamstrings, hip flexors, lower back, neck, calves always tight?
4. Do my knees come towards each other when I sit down?

How do I solve my Imbalance Problem?

QUESTION	ANSWER		PROBLEM	SOLUTION
	YES	NO		
1. Do my shoulders slouch and slump forward?			Weak Retractor Muscles, Overactive Chest	Strengthen Retractors*: Post. Deltoid, Teres Major Infraspinatous, Parts of Trapezius Stretch Chest, limit multiple exercises for chest
2. Does my butt stick out and does my lower back cave in? Is my lower back frequently tight or sore?			Weak Core, Genetic Influence Excessive Spinal Lordosis**	Strengthen Medius, Maximus in your Butt * Strengthen Abdominal wall – "Core" Stretch Hip Flexors, Lower Back, Quadriceps
3. Do my feet turn out when I walk, sit or stand? Do I walk like a duck?			Weak Gluteus Medius	Strengthen Medius, Stretch Calf Muscle
4. Do my knees knock together when I sit, stand, jump or squat?			Weak Abductor, Medius, Maximus Wide Pelvic Bone Placement	Strengthen Medius, Abductors, Maximus Stretch your IT band, Adductors
5. Does my neck stick forward like a turkey or duck?			This typically has to do with Bone Alignment	See a Chiropractor, Massage Therapist** Practice Holding Chin back and In*
6. Do my ankles cave in (this can either be one or both ankles)?			Weak Arches in your Foot	Strengthen Arch Get some Orthodic Inserts Stretch Peroneals

*Please refer to the Video on Muscular imbalances and THEIR SOLUTIONS

**Intervention of Chiropractic care would be helpful

RETRACTION!

I am a trainer known to say the word "Retract!" to my clients, repeatedly; sometimes as a gentle reminder, sometimes as a loud barking command. Either way, YOU MUST do it. You'll look weird and have problems if you don't!

What is it?

It enables you to activate the correct muscle throughout the range of movement, instead of resorting to the familiar (wrong) and overworked muscles. Retraction helps poor posture and strengthens weak muscles which aide in correct posture.

How do I do it?

Well, if drop your trapezius down, pull your posterior deltoid back and use your teres minor and major, rhomboids and infraspinatus doesn't mean anything to you, this might help:

Go up against a wall for starters, and plaster the back of your shoulders to the wall. THE MOST IMPORTANT THING is to...KEEP YOUR SHOULDERS DOWN!!! Then you will be correctly using the muscles that I want you to work. Do this exercise and hold it, then do it again. 3 sets of 15 reps if you need a number; hold for about 5 sec. As soon as you start shrugging up your shoulders, STOP and start over again.

Retraction Exercises

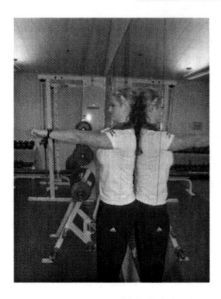 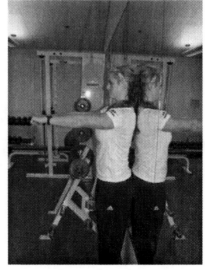

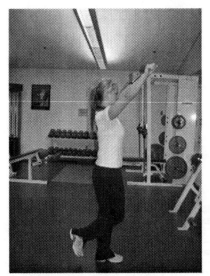 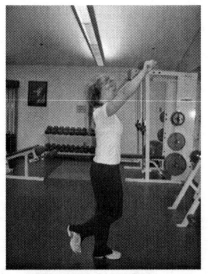

- EXTENDED PICTURES
- Go Up against a mirror and fully extend at the shoulder joint, forward
- Or, keep your arms fully extended upwards...

- RETRACTED PICTURES
- Then stick your chest out and flatten your shoulders up against the mirror
- Keep your shoulders down
- Then for the incline move, bring shoulders down

Muscles to use: Posterior Deltoid, Teres Minor/Major, Infraspinatus, Rhomboideus

Muscles NOT to use: The most overused muscle is the trapezius. The whole purpose of retraction is to teach you how to disengage your trapezius and to engage all the little guys that need to get worked.

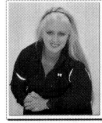

Christin's Tip!

If you constantly have soreness in your neck and shoulders, you need to be a MASTER of this exercise. One of the reasons may be because you are constantly putting stress and strain on your trapezius which directly connects to your shoulders and neck.

SHOES

Not all shoes are created equal! The proper shoes will spare you of injury and pain! Inserts are important as they prevent knee, lower back and hip pain.

Your fitness shoes should be:

- Lightweight
- Breathable
- Durable
- Comfortable
- Offer adequate support

Check out the recommendations on my website at: www.christinmcdowell.com.

To use or to not use inserts:

Take a look at the way you walk or stand in front of the mirror. If your ankle caves to the inside even just a little bit, you need them!

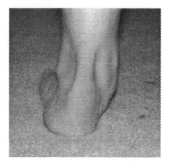

An ankle caving in to the right

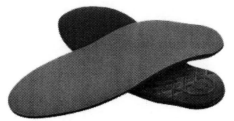

A good shoe insert

You can get them at any generic athletic store for around $20. I have found that the long flimsy inserts do not provide enough arch support, so I choose to go with the inserts with the hard plastic on the bottom.

Chapter 3

Men's Fitness

"Every man is the builder of a temple called his body. " Henry David Thoreau

Men! You are lucky. Be thankful for the day you were created as men, because unlike women, you have the ability to reach your fitness goals MUCH faster (that is, if you do it RIGHT). You have the ability to

1. Gain muscle faster
2. Lose body fat faster
3. Lower your blood pressure and your Resting Heart Rate faster
4. Not to mention the ability to be stronger, faster, and have more endurance.

If you pig out on cookies, you won't see it on your rear the next day. Oh yeah, and your fat is located underneath the muscle tissue, so even if you are overweight, you don't have cellulite riddled throughout your legs and ass. So NO WHINING. The one drawback is you usually die earlier! But do not fear, I am going to teach and tell you how to:

1. Live longer
2. Be healthier
3. Get stronger
4. Lose fat fast
5. Improve your cardiovascular system

Before we get started, I want to briefly outline the importance of weight training and doing cardio!

Intro to Weight Training

So it's probably pretty obvious that you need to build muscle mass right? Well if you didn't know here are some of the reasons why.

I have trained so many men who say, "Oh, I'm not trying to be a body builder, I'm just trying to get healthy!"... Let me get this out there, you couldn't look like a body builder unless you consume over 5-7,000 calories a day, train more than 4-5 days a week, eat SUPER clean and have the genetics of a well developed gorilla. Lifting weights, even lifting heavier weights,

IS NOT GOING TO MAKE YOU BECOME A BODY BUILDER! But it will make you healthier. Some benefits:

1. Your hormones were made to shed body fat with the increase of muscle mass
2. Your resting metabolic rate will dramatically increase, which means your ability to burn fat will be greatly enhanced
3. Your hemoglobin saturation will be enhanced, which means your ability to carry oxygen in your red blood cells will be greater
4. It will help stabilize your blood pressure
5. Stronger muscles
6. Better posture
7. Your endocrine (hormonal) system will respond well with numerous benefits including positive effects on testosterone
8. You will have a greater sense of euphoria
9. It will make your bones stronger and prevent the loss of minerals
10. Your resting heart rate will lower
11. You will have more self confidence with women, with yourself and with your peers
12. Delays the signs and appearances of aging

Intro to "Cardio"

Cardio is not just for women. It is for you too! HOWEVER, "Cardio" does not mean getting on some boring elliptical/cross trainer for 30 minutes and just plugging your way through... your bodies will respond MUCH better to a different stimulus that that! The workouts that I'm going to give you will make you work and get your heart rate up; using weights or a track!

Your body needs to be manipulated in nice and healthy ways if you really want to see the optimal changes in your heart rate, which is a direct reflection on the

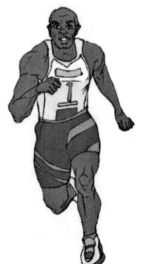

1. Strength of your heart
2. Blood pressure
3. Hemoglobin saturation

Cardio is the prolonged increase and elevation of your heart rate to a given stimulus. Here are some reasons why you need 'Cardio' in your life.

Some Benefits of Cardio

1. Longer life span
2. Lower blood pressure
3. Lower resting heart rate
4. Increased circulation
5. Prevention of disease
6. Enhances natural hormones
7. Healthier skin
8. Will release euphoric endorphins
9. Loss of body fat
10. Greater mobility and range of motion
11. Better circulation of nutrients and minerals
12. Improved overall sense of being

Manly Tips!

---

*"Always put your smile on. People will assume you are a crazy person
and won't mess with you"* Anon

---

1. Do not lift heavy weights if you have high blood pressure
2. Throw bouts of anaerobic intervals in your training (I'll explain that later)
3. Make sure to do some regular cardio
4. LIMIT or cut out alcohol, as it has an adverse affect on your hormones and progress with lifting; and everything else to do with your health
5. Eat healthy to live longer
6. Take GOOD multivitamins
7. Allow your body to heal by taking days off; that's how your muscle tissue grows
8. Eat real food, not meal replacement bars, fast food or bar food
9. Get enough sleep
10. Be consistent with your workouts

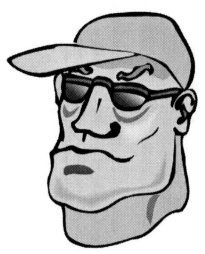

Testosterone!

What it is, why you need it and how to boost it NATURALLY

I'm sure you've all heard about the whole deal with the Rocket, the Juice (Bonds) and Big Mac? No… what do rockets, juice and big macs have to do with each other?!

Staying outta jail!

So what are ways you can boost your testosterone *naturally* without taking a trip to the slammer?

Anaerobic Training

One of the best ways to get in shape FAST is to use anaerobic training. The term anaerobic simply means 'without air-oxygen'. An example would be an all out 100% sprint for 50 meters, or doing a clean and jerk. There are many reasons why anaerobic training is so effective.

- Your cardiovascular system has to work hard to recover, which means that your resting heart rate, blood pressure and recovery time are all going to improve faster
- You will have a greater ability to burn fat for as the prime energy source at a higher intensity
- You will become faster and stronger-with more developed 'Type A' (fast twitch) muscle fibers

There any many things to consider with anaerobic training and how to use it to burn fat. You need to have a solid aerobic system before going all out, which is exactly what anaerobic training is! So don't go out there and start sprinting your heiny off after sitting on the couch for the past 10 years! It is important that anaerobic training is used by someone who is at Low Risk on the Assessment illustration (see chapter 2). You shouldn't attempt excessive sprints if you're just starting off or if you have high blood pressure. Build up a good base of aerobic conditioning first.

You are, of course, doing some anaerobic training every time you take a breath in to get ready for a squat, but that's quite a bit different from heavy duty sprinting that you would use with 100 meter and 200 meter runs! For now, if you are at high risk or overweight, you need to focus on BREATHING throughout your weight training and cardio.

Exercises such as using the medicine ball, sprinting on an elliptical or treadmill, are all examples of anaerobic training and will be included in the more advanced workout programs. I would only recommend using anaerobic training for healthy individuals strong enough to withstand the impact.

If you feel ready after 4-6+ months and do not have any risks factors, start off at 75-85% sprints and go from there. Do not do anaerobic sprints until you are fully ready and have built up a good aerobic base.

Training

Getting started

Common Terms and Vocab:

Set: How many times you complete the exercise, grouping

Reps: Repetition of exercise, e.g. Bicep Curl, 1,2,3,4,5,6,7,8= Reps, you do that 3x's and it's a Set!

SS: Superset: to do a set of 1 exercise then move on to the next!

Lever: The joint that moves the "Arm" of the Lever- i.e. your bicep and your forearm, so a biceps curl is a single lever movement

Compound Muscle Movement: A multi-dimensional movement that incorporates many muscles, e.g. Squat, Curl/Turn/Press, Plie

Auxiliaries/Auxiliary Training: Single lever movement, e.g. Single Leg Extensions, Biceps Curl, Back Row, etc.

Opposing Muscle Group: Muscles that are not directly related to the muscle you just worked e.g. Biceps Curl, then on to Triceps Extension, or your Hamstrings then your back

CV: Cardiovascular Work

LT CV: Light Cardio

WTS: Weights

CR: Core

WU: Warm UP

MD: Moderate intensity

LT: Light weight

PA: Physical Activity: These are things that just involve movement: raking the leaves, mowing the lawn, gardening, vacuuming, washing your car… etc. Or fun things like taking your kids to the park AND playing with them, Frisbee, golf, etc.

BDWT RX: Body weight exercises

JHR, J: Jack up the heart rate interval time! This will mean that after a set you will do a series of exercises to jack up your heart rate!

1. High knee Skips 25 Sec (see Exercise Reference examples in the back of the book)
2. High knees 25 Sec
3. Butt Kicks 25 Sec
4. Mountain Climbers 25 Sec

Interval: Alternating between hard and low intensities

Pool: Pool workouts are very important because they bring your heart rate up while bypassing the negative effects gravity can bring. There's something called 'increased thoracic pressure', which means because of the water pressure on the heart and lungs, your cardiovascular system will have to work harder than you think, though you may not feel it! So it's great for lowering blood pressure and sparing joints!

If you have high blood pressure:

Always make sure you are breathing regularly throughout all your exercises! Holding your breath creates a highly pressurized state in your body, so <u>breath regularly</u>! During weight training, inhale on the easy part and exhale on the hard part. Avoid heavy weight training until you get your blood pressure under control. Your focus should be on using lighter weight for higher reps.

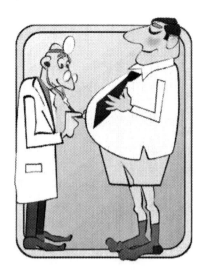

I have some great workouts that are made especially for people who are overweight and/or who have high blood pressure.

Training: If you are Obese or Overweight by 30lbs or more

Heavy weight training is one of the biggest mistakes I see with men and women who are severely overweight. Think about it! Your muscles are already working twice as hard because you are carrying around so much excess weight. You should focus on getting your heart rate up by just simply moving... your heart rate will climb up fast so take it easy. You will be the best judge on whether you need to slow down or take a break.

Using a heart rate monitor is also very important to make sure your heart rate doesn't get too high and so you can track your progress. Use the HRR formula in chapter 2 to calculate your heart rate. A good recommendation may be a 50-70% range. If you feel your heart rate is too easy or too hard, slow it down or speed it up. Focus on having longer workouts vs. more intense workouts.

Christin H. McDowell

Training Programs for Overweight Men

> *"I can't stop eating. I eat because I'm unhappy, and I'm unhappy because I eat. It's a vicious cycle. Now, if you'll excuse me, there's someone I'd like to get in touch with and forgive... myself."* Fat Bastard (The Spy who Shagged Me)

These programs are for you if you are just starting out and/or are overweight. It is going to be VERY important you do your cardio because your organs (especially your lungs and heart) need to get stronger and more efficient.   Think of your body as a car that has been sitting out in the cold and rain for many years and hasn't been driven. It needs some TLC and some cleaning before you expect it to run well...same goes for your body. Therefore, I am recommending you do about 2-4 weeks of steady state cardio before you jump into a holistic training program.

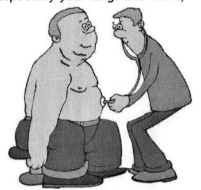

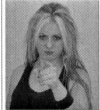

Christin's Rant!

Heavy weight training is one of the biggest mistakes I see with men and women who are severely overweight. Think about it!   Your muscles are already working twice as hard because you are carrying around so much excess weight. You should focus on getting your heart rate up by just simply moving... your heart rate will climb up fast so take it easy. You will be the best judge on whether you need to slow down or take a break. Steady state cardio means to exercise with your heart rate at a set range... (i.e workout at 110bts/min for 45 min, 3x/wk for two weeks).   This is important to help strengthen your heart steadily and safely.

A Heart Rate Monitor is also very important to make sure your heart rate doesn't get too high, and so you can track your progress. Use the HRR formula in chapter 2 to calculate your heart rate. A good recommendation may be a 50-70% range. If you feel your heart rate is too easy or too hard, slow it down or speed it up.

At this time, avoid intense workouts. Interval work should be limited; it will come later. Remember slow and steady is the key! Your focus should be as much on eating well and reducing caloric intake as it should be on working out. You can't go buck wild with your physical training, so go buck wild on eating right! (Make sure you get a copy of Healthy Dude Book!)

I have created a 7 day program which has Monday-Sunday labeled for training days. Adjust appropriately to your own schedule. (If the workout is too much or too little, you will know by the way your body feels, so change it accordingly). You can move on to Workout #2 when you feel ready.

Pool workouts will also be VERY important to you. They will help you get your heart rate up and move freely without feeling the negative effects of gravity! You'll feel like a million bucks when the workout's over too! (See page 123)

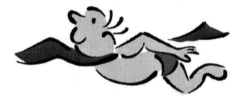

Program 1:   Severely overweight 50+lbs

Program 2:   Moderately overweight 30-50lbs; You have a lot of Existing Muscle Mass

Program 3:   Moderately overweight 30-50lbs; You don't have a lot of Existing Muscle Mass

Severely Overweight

Always follow what your body is saying. If you need to speed up, speed up and if you need to slow down or stop, do so!

7 Day Layout

Monday	Tuesday	Wednesday	Thursday	Friday	Saturday	Sunday
CV 30-40 Min	CV 5-10Min WRKT #1	OFF or LT Pool Wrkt	CV 30-40+ Min	CV 5-10 Min WRKT #1	OFF	Pool

Workout 1

Exercise	Sets	Reps	Weight		Reference #
Walk in Place:	2		BDWT		
High knees	2	6-10			J2
Butt Kicks	2	6-10			J3
Step Up Up Down Down	2	5-6 Each leg		Stage 1	L17
(On a small ledge)					
Side to Side Jumping Jack	2	5 Each leg			
(A Jumping Jack but walking)					
Walk 20 m	2	or 1 Min			
Knee Push Up	2	8-15	BDWT		C5
Sit Up Sit Down, Using a Chair	2	8-10	BDWT	Stage 2	L13
Crunches	2	10-15	BDWT		CR1
Walk in Place	2	30 Sec			
Chest Press Barbell or Machine	1-2	10-15	LT-MOD		C6
Dumbell Back Row	1-2	8-12	MOD	Stage 3	B4
Wide Grip Lat Pull Face	1-2	8	MOD		B5
Narrow Grip Lat Pull Away	1-2	10-12	LT		B6

Walking Punch	1-2	5 Each Arm	LT		S6
Walking Curls-	1-2	6 Each Arm			PB2
NOT on the Ball, <u>WALKING...</u>					
Finish with Walking		10-15Min+			
and/or				Stage 4	
Moving the Elliptical		5-15Min+			

Workout 2

Exercise	Sets	Reps	Weight		Reference #
Walk in Place ROUTINE:	1		BDWT		
1. High knees	1	6-10			J2
2. Butt Kicks	1	6-10			J3
3. Step Up Up Down Down	1	5-6 Each leg		Stage 1	L17
(On a small ledge)					
4. Side to Side Jumping Jack	1	5 Each leg			
(A Jumping Jack but walking)					
Walk 20 m	1	or 1 Min			
Knee Push Up	1	8-10			C5
Crunches	2	8-10		Stage 2	CR1
Up/Up Down Downs	2	5-6			CR10
(Upper Body, on Knees)					
Walk in Place Routine	1				
Bench Press Barbell	2	12-20	45+lbs, Easy-Mod		C12
DMBL Row	2	10-15	Mod		
Wide Grip Lat Pull Face	2	8	Mod		B5
Narrow Grip Lat Pull Away	2	10-12	LT	Stage 3	B6
Curl Turn Press	1-2	6-10	Mod		Bi2
Squats	1-2	10-12	BDWT		L13
Foot Step Up/Up Down Downs	2	5-8 Each leg	BDWT		L17
Walking -OR-		5-15Min+			
Moving the Elliptical					
CORE WORK		3-5 Min			CR-

Program 2

You're overweight and have a lot of existing muscle mass

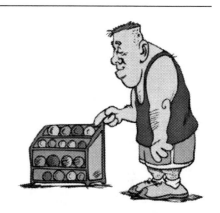

You need to focus on doing a lot of bodyweight exercises and high reps back to back; not using a ton of weight.

After you drop the first 15-20lbs, you can add more weight and advance to the 'Training for the Average Joe workout'.

7 Day Layout

Monday	Tuesday	Wednesday	Thursday	Friday	Saturday	Sunday
CV 5-10 Min WRKT #1	CV 45-60min	CV 45-60 Min or Pool	OFF	CV 5-10 Min WRKT #1	CV 45-60	Pool or OFF

Workout

Exercise	Sets	Reps	Weight		Reference #
Floor Push Ups	2	10-15	BDWT		C2
Barbell Back Row	2	15-20	45lbs		B1
Barbell Bench Press	2	15-20	45lbs	Stage 1	C12
Up Up Down Downs	2	5-8 Each Arm	BDWT		CR10
Triceps Dips	2	15	BDWT		Tri3
1min Elliptical Fast	2	1min			
JHR!!					J 1-4
45°Press	2	12-20	45-65lbs		C1
Full sit up	2	8-15	BDWT		CR5
Lat Pull Hands Face,	2	6-10	Mod	Stage 2	L5
Lat Pull Hands Away	2	8-12	LT		L6
Up Up Down Downs	2	5-6 Each Arm	BDWT		CR10
1min Fast Elliptical	2	1min			
Stair Stepper	2	30 Sec			
Squats	2	8-12	BDWT	Stage 3	L13
Squat Curl Turn Press	2	10-15	LT-Mod		L13,S3
Wide Leg Press	2	15-20	LT		L18
Narrow Leg Press	2	10-12	LT		L9
Treadmill	1	2-3 Min	Mod-Fast, Run		
Full sit up	1	8-10	BDWT	Stage 4	CR5
Crunch, Butt lift with Barbell	1	10	45lbs		CR11
Walking -OR-		5-15Min+			
Moving the Elliptical					

Program #2

You're overweight and don't have a lot of existing muscle mass

Your focus will be on a combination of muscle gain and the expenditure of calories. You will have a comprehensive program that focuses on the manipulation of your heart rate through various body weight and weighted exercises. Your program will also include spurts of cardiovascular exercises to increase your potential to burn fat. After you drop about 20lbs, increase the amount of weight and decrease the reps.   Some anaerobic training will also be incorporated. An example of this is the Average Joe Workout.

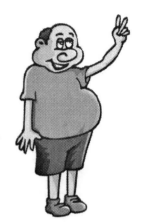

7 Day Layout

Monday	Tuesday	Wednesday	Thursday	Friday	Saturday	Sunday
CV 5-10 Min WRKT #1	CV 45-60min	OFF or POOL	CV 5-10 Min WRKT #1	CV 45-60min	Lifts-Whatever is not sore	Pool or OFF

Workout

	Sets	Reps	Weight		Reference #
Floor Push Ups	2	10-15	BDWT	Stage 1	C2
Barbell Back Row	2	15-20	45lbs		B1
Barbell Bench Press	2	15-20	45lbs		C12
Up Up Down Downs	2	5-8 Each Arm	BDWT		CR10
Triceps Dips	2	15	BDWT		T3
JHR!!				Stage 2	J 1-4
Barbell Chest Press	2	8-15	MOD		C12
Full sit up	2	8-15	BDWT		CR5
Barbell Back Row	2	8-12	45+lbs		B1
DMBL Back Row			20+lbs		B4
Lat Pull Hands Face	2	8-12	MOD		B5
Lat Pull Hands Away	2	5-6 Each Arm	MOD		B6
2 Min Elliptical	2	1min			
JHR!!				Stage 3	J 1-4
Incline DMBL Chest Press	2	8-10	25+LBS		C4
Curl Turn Press	2	6-8	15+/- LBS MOD		Bi2
Triceps Extension	2	8-12	15+/- LBS MOD		Tri2
Shrugs	2	12-20	HEAVY		S2
1min Elliptical				Stage 4	
Stair Stepper	2	30 Sec			
Wide Leg Press	2	15-20	MOD		L18
Narrow Leg Press	2	10-12	MOD		L9
Treadmill	1	2-3 Min	Mod-Fast, Run	Stage 5	
Full sit up	1	8-10	BDWT		CR5
Crunch, Butt lift with Barbell	1	10	45lbs		CR11
Walking -OR-		5-15Min+			
Moving the Elliptical					

Average Joe

What he should know and do about getting in shape!

"Train, say your prayers, and eat your vitamins" Hulk Hogan

The 'Average Joe' can be anyone from his mid 20's to his late 50's. Average Joe nowadays is a long way away from GI Joe! The Average Joes I see usually have quite a belly (lots of unhealthy fat stacked around the internal organs), drinks too much (bad for liver, kidneys, and general well being), eats way too much and exercises far too little. Average Joe is not as healthy as he should be and that's a problem.

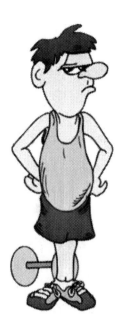

If this sounds like you, you need help a heck of a lot more than you think.   We now know that being overweight in your 40's can lead to mental challenges, cardiovascular disease, heart attacks, high blood pressure, diabetes, strokes and more. You MUST do something about your health and fitness, and it starts today, right now.

You need a game plan.

- Choose days out of the week you can commit to working out. I recommend you start by hitting 4 days a week. Too many people say they don't have time to work out, then change their minds after the first heart attack...so let's turn that around and MAKE time NOW.   There are 24hrs in a full day, so commit at least one of them to your health.

- Start eating *and* drinking healthy right now, read Healthy Dude Book and start applying it to your life.

<u>Training:</u> Where to Start...

1. Assessment: Check your weight now then set a target weight. Measure your waist girth as well. This will be around your belly button. Track these measurements down on your computer or a piece of paper that you will be able see often to help you with your motivation. You should be able to lose 1-2lbs/week IF you do everything right. If you aren't perfect, you should still be able to hit 1 lb a week. If you don't lose at least a pound per week, you will need to reevaluate what you are doing, because it's wrong... most likely it's coming from your eating. In order to lose 1 lb of fat you need to burn 3,500 calories. 3500 calories/7 days is only 500 calories per day, which might be your afternoon snack and a brisk jog, so dropping 500 calories/day is definitely doable.

2. The next thing you need to do is figure out your **Risk Factors** if you have any. Refer to Chapter 2, and create either a THR or HRR. This will make sure you are starting off safely with your heart. Chances are your HR prescription might be too easy, but you should still stay with it until you feel absolutely ready. This might be in 1 week or 3 months, it totally depends on your level of fitness and cardiovascular health.

3. If you have problems with your knees, lower back or neck, you need to do a muscular imbalance assessment and see what exercises you should do. (Chapter 2)

4. Tell a friend about your goals and ask them to harass the hell out of you to help you stay accountable. You can also go to TrishaStewart.com ask me for help. I am here for you! The MOST important thing is that you do THIS, and that you start TODAY. Not tomorrow, not next week, not when your boss gets back, not next month when your kid finally heads off to school, TODAY.

So here is an optimal 7 day layout that is HIGHLY achievable, so don't make excuses. You can switch around the days of course, but nothing else.

PA means Physical Activity. This would include playing golf, doing yard work, sex, and anything else that gets your heart rate up. Having an active lifestyle is important to your health and well being. If it is lacking in physical activities, come up with ways to make it more interesting, e.g. going hiking, sledding with the kids, fishing, canoeing, diving, biking, skiing, bowling etc.

If you're already in decent shape, I have included an Advanced Average Joe workout, 1&2. I would still start off with the Average Joe workout. All you average Joes, progress onto the Advanced 1 & 2 workouts when you feel ready. Use your own discretion when you feel you need to move on to the harder workout...everyone's different. When you've finished with the Advanced Average Joes workouts, and feel they're too easy, you can progress to the Super Joe Workout.

Average Joe 7 Day Layout and Workouts

Monday	Tuesday	Wednesday	Thursday	Friday	Saturday	Sunday
WKRT 15-20 CV	45-60 CV	OFF or POOL	WRKT 15-20 CV	45-60 CV	OFF or POOL	PA!!

Average Joe Workout

	Sets	Reps	Weight		Reference #
Floor Push Ups	1	10-15	BDWT		C2
Barbell Back Row	1	15-20	45lbs		B1
Barbell Bench Press	1	15-20	45lbs	Stage 1	C12
Up Up Down Downs	1	5-8 Each Arm	BDWT		CR10
Triceps Dips	1	15	BDWT		Tri3
JHR!!	1				J 1-4
Barbell Chest Press	2	8-10	MOD		C12
Barbell Back Row	2	8-12	45+lbs		B1
DMBL Back Row	2	8-12	25+lbs		B4
Incline Chest Press	2	6-10	MOD-Heavier	Stage 2	C4
Lat Pull Hands Face	2	6-8	Heavier		B5
Lat Pull Hands Away	2	8-12	MOD		B6
1 Min Elliptical and JHR!!	1				J 1-4
Curl Turn Press	2	6-8	15+/- LBS MOD		Bi2
Triceps Extension	2	8-12	15+/- LBS MOD	Stage 3	T2
Shrugs	2	12-20	HEAVY		S2
Up Up Down Downs	2	5-8 Each Arm	BDWT		CR10
1min Elliptical	1				
Stair Stepper	2	30 Sec		Stage 4	
Wide Leg Press	2	15-20	MOD		L18
Narrow Leg Press	2	10-12	MOD		L9
Treadmill	1	2-3 Min	Mod-Fast, Run		
Full sit up	1	8-10	BDWT	Stage 5	CR5
Crunch, Butt lift with Barbell	1	10	45lbs		CR11

The <u>Advanced Average Joe</u> Workouts 1-2

These workouts are for men who consider themselves in good physical shape. There are a lot of bodyweight exercises, supersets with anaerobic intervals and weight training. Keep in mind that to make the workout hard, minimize your breaks! You can increase the intensity of the workouts by adding weight and reps. If your focus is on getting bigger, increase the amount of weight...otherwise just increase the amount of reps.

I have included two workouts:

- Workout 1: Upper Body
- Workout 2: Lower Body

Note: you can supplement exercises from either workout based on how your body is feeling

7 Day Layout and Workouts

Monday	Tuesday	Wednesday	Thursday	Friday	Saturday	Sunday
WKRT 1 5-10 Min CV	45-60 CV and/or Pool	WRKT 2 5-10 Min CV	OFF Or Sports	LIFT what's not sore LT CV 20-30 min	OFF or POOL Hiking etc	PA!!

Advanced Average Joe Workout #1

	Sets	Reps	Weight		Reference #
Floor Push Ups (ON FEET)	1	10-15	BDWT		C5
Barbell Back Row	1	15-20	45lbs		B1
Barbell Bench Press	1	15-20	45lbs	Stage 1	C12
Up Up Down Downs	1	5-8 Each Arm	BDWT		CR10
Triceps Dips	1	15	BDWT		Tri3
Elliptical Sprint	1	45 Sec			
JHR!!	1				J 1-4
Physioball Dumbell Chest Press	2	8-10	MOD		C8
Barbell Back Row	2	8-12	25+lbs		B1
Dumbell Incline Chest Press	2	6-10	MOD-Heavier	Stage 2	C4
Floor-to-Bench Up Up Down Downs	2	6-8	Heavier		CR10
Shrugs	2	10-15	Heavy		S2
Elliptical Sprint	3	45 Sec			
JHR!!	1				J 1-4
Curl Turn Press	2	6-8	MOD		Bi2
Triceps Extension	2	8-12	MOD		Tri2
Triceps Dips	2	12-20	BDWT		Tri3
Double Arm Biceps Curl NOT ON BALL	2	12-20	LT-MOD	Stage 3	PB2
Shoulder Rasies-0,45,90°	2	6 Each Way	LT-MOD		S1
Posterior Deltoid	2	6-12	LT-MOD		S5
Elliptical Sprints	1-2				
Core:					
Physioball Crunch	2	15			PB3
Barbell Crunch, Butt lift	2	10-15			CR11
Side Crunch	2	10-20			CR9

Advanced Average Joe Workout #2

	Sets	Reps	Weight		Reference #
Elliptical Warm Up	2 min				
Running Sprints	5	20-50 Meters or (.12)	90% Intensity	Stage 1	
Run	2	400M or (.25)	80% Intensity		
Wtd Step Up	2	6-8 Each Leg	Mod-Heavy		L17
Barbell Wide Squat	2	8-12	Mod	Stage 2	L13
Wide Leg Press	2	8-12	Mod-Heavy		L18
Narrow Leg Press	2	10-12	Mod		L9
Elliptical Sprints	2-3	20-30 Sec		Stage 3	
Stair Stepper Sprint	2-3	20-30 Sec			
Auxiliaries:					
Quad Extension	1-2	8-12	Mod-Heavy		L14
Hamstring Curl	1-2	8-12	Mod-Heavy		L6
Abductor	1-2	12-15	Mod-Heavy	Stage 4	L1
Adductor	1-2	10-15	Mod		L2
Calves	1-2	12	Mod-Heavy		L20
CORE	5 min	Your Choice!			CR-

Super Jock!

"When the Boogeyman goes to sleep every night, he checks his closet for Chuck Norris." Anon

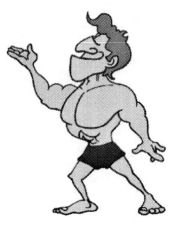

You have arrived! You are at the level of fitness you want to be...or are you?? Let these workouts challenge your level of fitness and inspire you to become even fitter!

Super Jock 7 Day Layout and Workouts

Monday	Tuesday	Wednesday	Thursday	Friday	Saturday	Sunday
WKRT 1	45-60 Sprints Plyometrics	WRKT 2	OFF	Combo Train Workouts 1 & 2	POOL Hiking etc	Off/ PA!!

Workout #1

	Sets	Reps	Weight		Reference #
400m Warm Up Run				Stage 1	
Sprints 7x 100m	1	7	100%		
Med Ball Throws:					
Chest Throw	2	8			M1
Behind the Head	2	8			M4
Barbell Squat (then) Jump	2	12	Mod	Stage 2	L5
Narrow Dumbell Squat	2	8-10	Heavy		L8
Quad Extension	2	12-15	Mod		L14
Hamstring Curl	2	12-15	Mod		L6
Double Leg Jumps	2	15			L19
Bike Sprints	2	1 min 20 Sec on 20 Sec Off			
Full Sit Up to Jump w/ Medball	2	8			CR12
Up Up Down Down's	2	6 Each			CR10
Mtn Climbers	2	25 Sec			J4
Shrug, Curl Turn Press	2	8	Mod-Heavy	Stage 3	S2, Bi2
Lat Pull Narrow	2	8	Heavy		B5
Lat Pull Wide	2	12	Mod		B6
Push Up Pop's	2	15			C10
Body Weight Pull Ups:	2				
Narrow/Neutral	2	8+			
Away & Facing	2	6+			
Elliptical Sprints	2	45 Sec	Hard-100%		

Negative Biceps Curls	2	6 Each	Heavy		Bi3
Double Arm Band Curl	2	25	Mod		Bi1
Heavy Triceps Ext	2	8-10	Heavy	Stage 4	Tri2
Triceps Dips	2	25+	Bdwt or Wtd		Tri3
400m Run					

WORKOUT #2

	Sets	Reps	Weight		Reference #
Elliptical Sprints 5min		25 Sec Sprint, <25Sec			
4x200m Run Fast				Stage 1	
Push Up Pop Offs	2	15	BDWT		C10
Barbell Back Row	2	25	BDWT		B1
Chest Press	3-5	6-12	Mod-Heavy		C12
Incline Dumbell Chest Press	3-5	6-8	Heavy		C4
Floor Up Up Down Downs	3	6 Each	BDWT	Stage 2	CR10
Triceps Dips	3-5	20+	BDWT or Wtd		Tri3
Up Up Down Downs on Bosu	3	6 Each	BDWT		CR10
Plyo's: Double Leg Jumps	2	12	BDWT or Wtd		L19
(onto box or bench)			with Medball		
Alt Stationary Lunge jump on Bosu	2	12	BDWT or Wtd	Stage 3	L16
JHR!!	2				J 1-4

Single Arm Dumbell Back Row	3-5	8-10	Heavy		B4
Double Machine back Row	3-5	6-12	Mod-Heavy		B9
Band Back Row	3-5	15-25	LT-MOD		B2
Shrugs	3-5	8-12	Heavy		S2
Upright Rows	3	6-10	Mod	Stage 4	S8
Shoulder Raises: Front, Middle, Side	2-3	5-6 Each	LT-MOD		S1
Floor Up Up Down Downs	2-3	6 Each	BDWT		CR10
Posterior Deltoid	2-3	5-10	LT-MOD		S5
30 Sec Sprint Elliptical	3				
2 min on Elliptical or 800 Meter Run					
Core:				Stage 5	
Physioball Crunch	2	15			PB3
Barbell Crunch, Butt lift	2	10-15			CR11
Side Crunch	2	10-20			CR9

Try to go as fast as you can from one exercise to the next, with little or no break time until you get to the end of the sequence.

Skinny Beans

I'm not fat. I'm skinny and I want to get BIG!

"You know, like nunchuku skills, bow hunting skills, computer hacking skills... Girls only want boyfriends who have great skills ..." Kip, Nippy D's Brother

What you need to focus on:

1. **Stuffing your face full of healthy food**
2. **Stuff your face again....**
3. **Lift 'til you feel like puking!**

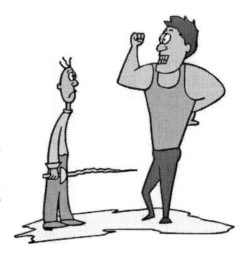

Whatever you feel is a lot of food, make it a TON. You MUST stuff your face. I repeat, stuff your face! Get some good quality mass gainer shakes, eat a lot of complex carbohydrates, fruit and vegetables. Protein is important, but carbohydrates are just as important, if not more. Try to lift 3-4x/wk and make sure your muscles have adequately recovered from their workout before you train them again.

Big shocker here; if your muscles haven't recovered, work different muscles!

- If your muscles recover within 1 day, you need to lift heavier weight and achieve greater muscular breakdown
- Don't train any muscle group more than 2x/wk, otherwise you won't allow them to heal properly
- Take good quality vitamins and antioxidants, they will help your cells repair faster. Go to www.trishastewart.com for recommendations on supplements
- Get enough sleep and rest
- Limit your cardio

Skinny Beans 7 Day Layout and Workouts

Monday	Tuesday	Wednesday	Thursday	Friday	Saturday	Sunday
WKRT 1	OFF	5-10 Min CV WRKT 2	OFF Or Sports	5-10 Min CV WRKT 3	PA	PA OFF

Workout #1

For Bench & Back Do warm Up sets	Sets	Reps	Weight	Reference #
Barbell Bench Press or 45	3-5	6-10	Mod-Heavy	C12
Barbell Back Row	3-5	10-15	Mod-Heavy	B1
Dumbell Back Row	3-5	8-12	Heavy	B4
Shrugs	3-5	12-20	Heavy	S2
Dumbell Incline Bench	3-5	6-10	Mod-Heavy	C4
Dumbell Fly	2-3	8-12	MOD	PB4
Curl Turn Press	3-4	6-10	MOD	Bi2
Upright Rows	2-3	8-12	LT-MOD	S8
Shoulder Rasies-0,45,90°	2-3	6 Each way	LT-MOD	S1
Posterior Deltoid	2-3	6-10	LT-MOD	S6

Workout #2

	Sets	Reps	Weight	Reference #
Lat Pull Down Face	3-4	6-8	Heavy	B5
Lat Pull Down Away	3-4	12	Mod	B6
Pull Ups:				
Away	3	Max		
Neutral	3	Max		
Face	3	Max		
Alt. Biceps Curls (Not on Pball)	3	8-12	Heavy	PB2
Negative Curls	3	6	Heavy	Bi3
Triceps Extension	3	6-8	Heavy	Tri2
Triceps Dips	3	12-20	BDWT	Tri3

Workout #3

	Sets	Reps	Weight	Reference #
Wide Leg Press	3-5	8-12	Heavy	L18
Narrow Leg Press	3-5	10-15	Mod-Heavy	L9
Wtd Step Up	3-5	6-10	Heavy	L17
Narrow Squat	3-5	8-21	Mod-Heavy	L8
Auxiliaries:				
Quad Extension	2-3	12-15	Mod-Heavy	L14
Hamstring Curl	2-3	12-15	Mod-Heavy	L6
Abductor	2-3	12-15	Mod-Heavy	L1
Adductor	2-3	12-15	Mod-Heavy	L2
Calves	2-3	12-15	Heavy	L20

So you have a whole set of workouts for your weight and level of fitness.

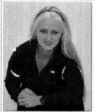

Christin's Tip!
Remember, men respond well to weight training because of the way their bodies are made. Always incorporate it into your program, even if you have a hard time of gaining mass, or if you don't want any added mass. Weight training can do anything for you; lean you down, add mass, shape your body and more!

Remember:

1. Supplement with a good multivitamin and add extra antioxidants with your new program. Your body will need more vitamins and minerals to repair tissue damage and replenish stores. You'll spare yourself injury, burnout, have more energy and feel better.

2. Take rest days! Rest days are necessary in order for your body to recover from intense exercise. Don't fall into the trap of over training or over extending your body early in your training program. You won't lose as much body fat, gain as much muscle or have as much fun if you do.

3. But just as important... don't convince yourself that you need to rest your body when all you really want is to avoid working out! In other words, DON'T BE LAZY! Your body will let you know when it needs rest; you'll know the difference.

4. Change it up! Find different ways you can challenge your body to adapt to a new stimulus. This will prevent plateaus, stimulate fat loss and keep you interested.

5. Remember, if you ain't changing, you be doin' something wrong. You CANNOT go wrong with all the information and programs I have designed specifically for where you're at right now. So, there are no excuses as to why you can't have the body you want. Get it!

Chapter 5

Women's Fitness

"No matter who you are, no matter what you do, you absolutely, positively do have the power to change." Bill Phillips

A Word to Women...

Ladies, your bodies are waaay different from men's. (Duh!) It almost always takes longer to see gains or losses in any category of fitness, save flexibility and don't even get me started with the diet. There are many reasons for this unfortunate phenomenon... You have:

- less existing muscle mass
- your hormones protect your organs through preserving body fat
- your hormones promote the storage of body fat and thus your metabolic rate and your potential to burn energy throughout the day is already significantly lower

This simply means that the journey to achieving your fitness goals might be challenging but it is 100% doable if you train smart, effective and proactively.

There are several things you MUST take into account if you want to come become a shapely, fit woman.

1. You MUST train for your body type
2. You MUST do things you possibly hate

For an example, I hate long distance running. It bores me to tears! BUT, long distance running is the exact thing I need to change my body and bring it to the next level.

I am going to cover all the steps, jumps and hurdles you must go through to get the body you want. There are no diet pills, diets or surgeries that will make you fit. There are NO quick fixes! To bring about change, you must be active, effective, educated and persistent. If anyone tries to sell you differently, it's a hoax. So prepare yourself for the TRUTH about how to train and get amazing results!

I am going to tell you my **Woman's Training Philosophy** and correct some common misconceptions about exercising! Hopefully I will answer some of the questions you may have concerning cardio and weight training, and will have enlightened you on how to further maximize your time exercising.

Training Philosophy

You must train for your body type. The majority of women fall into 2 categories:

1. Women with fat accumulation around their abdomen (Android Fat Displacement)
2. Women with fat distribution to the butt and thigh (Gynoid Fat Displacement)

Occasionally I see women with both, so if that's you, you should mix and match from both the Android and Gynoid training regimes. Programs for both body types are covered in depth.

Everybody asks:

*   "How much weight training should I do?"
*   "How much cardio should I do and at what intensity?"
*   "Should I do cardio first or weight training?"

The answer is a little complicated... so put on your hard hats and listen up!

"Weight" training is simply using an overload on your body to achieve muscular breakdown. This is why you get sore; your muscles get torn on a microscopic level.

"Weight" training is important because it:

*   increases your bone density
*   strengthens your muscles
*   increases your resting metabolic rate and your metabolism
*   minimally strengthens your organs, heart, lungs etc., because of the pressure put on the cardiovascular system
*   reduces painful problems associated with the lower back, shoulders, neck, etc.

Now I say "weight" training, because you don't necessarily have to use weights to have this kind of an impact! Having weight means having an **overload**. You can **overload** your system WITHOUT doing weight training... i.e. USING YOUR OWN BODYWEIGHT!! Imagine being 30lbs overweight... go pick up a 30lb dumbbell and see how your body feels after just 1 min of carrying that thing around...hurts huh?? That's the amount of pressure your body endures day in and day out! So the last thing we need to do is pile on more weight as using your own bodyweight will suffice.

YOU CAN also manipulate your Cardio to have pretty much the same effect as weight training! Because weight training is simply the breakdown of muscle tissue, you can achieve the same result with intense cardiovascular training (such as sprints, long distance running, swimming, dance, ballet and sports). Try it! If you're trying to gain muscle SIZE, that's a bit different...but there aren't many women who are trying to do that...if you are, then pure lifting is definitely for you. (Check out Men's Fitness: I'm skinny and I want to get BIG!)

If DONE CORRECTLY, learning how to manipulate, change and enhance your cardiovascular training will have near double the positive effects as weight training. And hopping on the elliptical for 20mins doesn't cut it! There's no change, no manipulation and no alteration... in order to achieve the desired effect, you have to constantly **CHANGE, PROGRESS AND ENHANCE your cardio**. Here's why!

Manipulating cardiovascular work is the key to changing your body fat, leaning down and living longer.

Cardio:

- burns fat
- strengthens your organs and muscles
- enhances your balance
- improves the oxidation of red blood cells
- enriches and saturates your blood with more oxygen
- improves your resting heart rate and blood pressure
- reduces risk of diabetes and CVD
- helps prevents obesity
- improves quality of mind

So start implementing...

- running sprints
- running Long distance
- swimming Sprints
- swimming Long Distance
- biking Sprints
- biking Long Distance
- dancing
- kick Boxing
- plyometrics
- medball work

- fast walks
- walk uphill
- walk Uphill with weighs

...into your workouts! They'll shape your body and burn a TON of calories.

So, I'm not saying throw out the weight training; just focus on improving your fitness by the variety and intensity of cardiovascular work. Your muscles, heart, lungs and hormones will thank you.

Weight training can be a great tool for those who have difficulty moving such as the elderly, injured and astronauts! (If you _are_ an astronaut, email me for your zero gravity workouts!!) ::::just kidding::::

WRAP UP

Maximize and manipulate your cardio first and foremost, use plyometrics, bands and body weight exercises, swimming, biking, and stair stepper for extra sculpting.

On to Misconceptions!

1. Why "Cardio Zone" and "Fat Burning Zone" Don't Matter

It's all explained in chapter 2!

2. Protein

The hype these days is about protein, protein, protein! Did you know that protein is just like a carb or fat calorie? If it doesn't get used, it will be stored as fat! That's right! There is no difference; if you eat more than you need, your body will store protein as fat. This is why having balance and variety in your diet is all important. Everything you need to know about nutrition can be found in Trisha Stewart's book 'Healthy Tart'.

3. Working Out 2-3x/wk is Enough

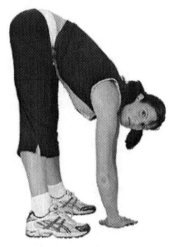

Not so. If you want to live longer and keep your heart healthy, then working out 3x/wk is the MINIMUM requirement. For sustained WEIGHT LOSS, the accepted recommendation is 1 HR of cardio, MOST DAYS OF THE WEEK. That's right, 1 HR of solid cardio just about every day.

"1 HR!! I can't do that!!" It's ok! Start off with less of a contribution and work your way up. It's fine to bounce around and do different modes of cardiovascular training, and it's even ok to split it into 20/20/20 or 45, 30 minute increments. The point is to keep your heart rate up for an hour. Don't stop and watch TV half way through it, keep working! It takes a while for the body to adjust to the stimulus of exercise, so keep workin!

If you're just starting out, it's ok to take small breaks, but as you progress in your fitness, cut out the breaks! I strongly recommend light interval training after a few months of steady state heart rate training, i.e., 45 min of 112bts/min exercise.

4. Why being Sore isn't always a good thing

You don't want to be constantly sore, and the sign of a good workout, DOESN'T mean that you are sore! A good workout will leave you exhausted and tight, but not so sore you are limping. I see women who are trying to lose body fat talking how they're too sore to do anything! That ladies, is contrary to what we want to have happen.

Movement burns fat. If you can't move, you ain't burning fat.

Womanly Tips

"Simplifying your life gives you more time for what you really do want time and energy for (like exercising, or reading, or taking a class)." Kathy Gates

1. Train for your body type
2. Manipulate and maximize your cardio
3. Do body weight exercises
4. Eat right!
5. Be patient and listen to your body
6. Get adequate sleep
7. Take time out for yourself
8. Take rest days
9. Get an occasional massage
10. Drink lots of water
11. Take the right multi-vitamin and antioxidants

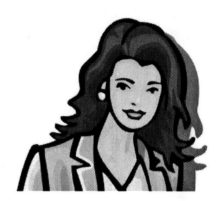

Common Terms and Vocab

- **Set**: How many times you complete the exercise, grouping
- **Reps**: Repetition of exercise, e.g. Bicep Curl, 1,2,3,4,5,6,7,8= reps, you do that 3x's and it's a Set
- **SS**: SuperSet: to do a set of 1 exercise then move on to the next
- **Lever**: The joint that moves the "arm" of the Lever- e.g. your bicep and your forearm, so a biceps curl is a single lever movement
- **Compound Muscle Movement**: A multi-dimensional movement that incorporates many muscles, e.g.: Squat, Curl turn Press, Plie
- **Auxiliaries/Auxiliary Training**: Single lever movement, e.g.: single leg extensions, biceps curl, back Row, etc.
- **Opposing Muscle Group**: Muscles that are not directly related to the muscle you just worked e.g.: biceps curl, then on to triceps extension, or your hamstrings then your back
- **CV:** Cardiovascular Work
- **LT** : Light Cardio, Weights
- **WTS**: Weights
- **CR:** Core
- **WU:** Warm UP
- **PA:** Physical Activity: These are things that involve movement: raking the leaves, mowing the lawn, gardening, vacuuming, washing your car...etc. Or fun things like taking your kids to the park AND playing with them, Frisbee, golf, etc.
- **BDWT RX:** Body weight exercises
- **JHR, J:** Jack up the heart rate interval time! This will mean that after a set you will do a series of exercises to jack up your heart rate! See **J** Exercise Reference Section.
    1. High Knee Skips 25 Sec
    2. High Knees 25 Sec
    3. Butt Kicks 25 Sec
    4. Mountain Climbers 25 Sec
- **Pool:** There's something called 'increased thoracic pressure' which means that because of the water pressure on your heart and lungs; your organs are really working even though the exercising doesn't feel hard. It's a great way of lowering your blood pressure without the negative effects gravity can bring!

Severely Overweight

Programs, Timelines, Advice and Encouragement!

"If I punched every b*tch who called me fat, it would be dead b*tches all up and down the highway." Star Jones

OK, you're severely overweight but you've decided enough is enough and you're seeking some good advice. That's the first step and I'm glad you ended up here, because together we can turn this around. I'm not going to try and convince you it's gonna be easy because it ain't. You have some unique challenges which you have to face head on! Number 1!!! You have to... have to... get your eating under control. Get Trisha Stewart's book 'Healthy Tart' to understand what's going on inside you and what you need to do to correct it. Doing all the exercises in the world won't help significantly unless you control your eating.

We are going to undertake a series of exercises, both in and out of the pool, which will be done in conjunction with your new eating regime, as set out in Healthy Tart. When you're done, you'll be a new person; healthier, fitter and a whole lot lighter.

Where to begin:

1. Set up a 7 Day Plan that you can follow
2. Get a Heart Rate monitor
3. Journal your emotions and thoughts with your eating and workouts
4. Monitor your progress by weighing yourself every 1-2 weeks
5. Check your blood pressure at least 1x/month

Heart Rate Monitor:

Using a heart rate monitor is also very important to make sure your heart rate doesn't get too high and so you can track your progress. Use the HRR formula in chapter 2 to calculate your heart rate. A good recommendation may be a 50-70% range. If you feel your heart rate is too easy or too hard, slow it down or speed it up. Focus on having longer workouts vs. more intense workouts.

Start off slow and easy, then up your workouts so you can go longer and longer. After that, you can start increasing the intensity of your workouts. I will provide 2 workouts for you as examples of a very low intensity and a moderate intensity. When you feel you are ready to increase the intensity of your workouts, you can progress on to training for your body type using either the Android or Gynoid workout programs. Start at the 'Beginner' level. You should also have definite improvements in your weight loss, blood pressure and resting heart rate before you advance on.

Using the pool as a mode of exercise will be VERY important to you. The pool will help you be able to get your heart rate up without feeling the negative effects that gravity has on your body. You will be able to move more and feel great! All the pool workouts start on page 123. Choose which best suits you; it doesn't matter if you can't swim, I have workouts for all levels and abilities!

Training Programs and Specifics

It is going to be VERY important you do your cardio because your organs (especially your lungs and heart) need to get stronger and more efficient.   Think of your body as a car that has been sitting out in the cold and rain for many years and hasn't been driven. It needs some TLC and some cleaning before you expect it to run well...same goes for your body. Therefore I am recommending you do about 2-4 weeks of steady state cardio before you jump into a holistic training program.

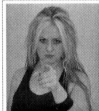

Christin's Rant!

Too many women believe that weight training is the key to weight loss. IT'S NOT!!! Cardio, Cardio, Cardio!!!!

Think about it! Your muscles are already working twice as hard because you are carrying around so much excess weight. You should focus on getting your heart rate up by just simply moving... your heart rate will climb up fast so take it easy. You will be the best judge on whether you need to slow down or take a break.

Steady state cardio means to exercise with your heart rate at a set range... (i.e. workout at 110bts/min for 45 min, 3x/wk for two weeks). This is important to help strengthen your heart steadily and safely.

At this time, avoid intense workouts. Interval work should be limited, it will come later. Remember slow and steady is the key! Your focus should be as much on eating well and reducing caloric intake as it should be on working out. You can't go crazy with your physical training, so go 'nuts' about eating right!

So here's your 7 day program...if it feels too much or too little, step it up or down accordingly. You can move on to Workout #2 when you feel ready to make your workouts a little more challenging.

7 Day Layout and Workouts

Monday	Tuesday	Wednesday	Thursday	Friday	Saturday	Sunday
CV 30-40 Min	CV 5-10Min WRKT #1	OFF or Pool WRKT	CV 30-40+ Min	CV 5-10 Min WRKT #1	OFF	Pool

Workout #1

<u>Exercise</u>	<u>Sets</u>	<u>Reps</u>	<u>Weight</u>		<u>Reference #</u>
Walk in Place:	2		BDWT		
High knees	2	6-10			J2
Butt Kicks	2	6-10		Stage 1	J3
Step Ups (On a small ledge)	2	5-6 Each leg			L17
Jumping Jack	2	5 Each leg			
Walk 20 m	2	or 1 Min			
Knee Push Up	2	8-15	BDWT		C5
Sit Up Sit Down, Using a Chair	2	8-10	BDWT	Stage 2	L13
Crunches	2	10-15	BDWT		CR1
Walk in Place	2	30 Sec			

Christin H. McDowell

Chest Press Barbell or Machine	1-2	10-15	LT-MOD		C6
Dumbell Back Row	1-2	8-12	MOD		B4
Wide Grip Lat Pull Face	1-2	8	MOD	Stage 3	B5
Narrow Grip Lat Pull Away	1-2	10-12	LT		B6
Walking Punch	1-2	5 Each Arm	LT		S6
Walking Curls- NOT on the Ball, WALKING...	1-2	8-10 Each Arm			PB2
Finish with Walking		10-15Min+			
and/or				Stage 4	
Moving the Elliptcal		5-15Min+			

Android Women

Android apple is fat in trunk and abs

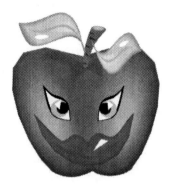

I admit it; I'm jealous. You Android women can get away with a few extra pounds. You have the bulk of your bodyfat around your belly, chest and some on your arms. Your legs tend to always be skinny now matter how much weight you gain. Thus, in the fitness and exercise world, you are condoned as 'apple' shaped women!

If you gain weight, you can get by with wearing some cute, tiny shorts and a nice big shirt; lucky for you, an easy cover up! But wait! There's more!

The Pro's

1. You can look good in short shorts!
2. You normally have a nice, large chest-then envy of many girls!
3. You will SEE results faster than a Gynoid woman.
4. You will change fast if you stick with your exercise program.

The Con's

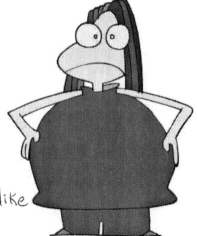

1. Fat accumulation around the abdomen means there's more pressure and fat near your internal organs. This is a bad thing and is more dangerous than having gynoid (pear) fat displacement.
2. If you gain a lot of weight, you end up looking like you're pregnant!

Training as an Androidian

Your Training Rules

- You, my friends, must build up <u>some</u> muscle mass and strengthen your back, arms and chest through body weight exercises, and weight training (make sure your main focus is still on cardio, page 57). If you already have a lot of muscle mass, focus on body weight exercises only: e.g. pushups and core work.
- Do cardio intervals during weight lifting.
- Make extra sure you know how to 'Retract' when weight training your upper body. Chances are you overuse your shoulders a lot because of having centrally located body fat.
- Minimize weight training for your legs; do cardio, sprints, and high rep body weight exercises instead. Your legs are already pretty strong if you're carrying extra weight in your belly!
- Clean out your intestines with Trisha Stewart's Healthy Tart 30 Day Detox program. Chances are there's a lot of toxic build up in and around your intestines and organs due to the excess abdominal fat. If you're pooping 2-3x/day you'll know 'the cleanse' is working!
- You'll probably experience radical changes at first, then plateau. Therefore, you must be diligent about eating well, Healthy Tart style, maybe with a little more added protein because of lifting more. When you are about 20-30lbs from your goal weight, limit all weight training. Start training like a Gynoid; lots of cardio and some bodyweight exercises: high knees, butt kicks, mountain climbers, full sit up to jumps, sprints, etc., and more abdominal work: sit ups, butt lifts, bosu crunches, bosu side crunches etc.
- Finish it out! Don't settle for just having a smaller waist or a small gut. Get rid of that 'thing' once and for all and don't settle for less. You deserve it!
- Be happy! Your results will come FAST if you follow the guidelines.
- Get in the Pool!!!!! All the pool workouts start on page 123. Choose which best suits you; it doesn't matter if you can't swim, I have workouts for all levels and abilities!

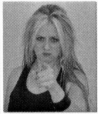 ## Christin's Rant!

I have heard every excuse you can imagine about why you can't get into the pool! "I look like a beached whale!!", "Everyone will laugh at me", "I suck at swimming", and many more.
What I say is "GET OVER IT!!!, Most people are too busy worrying about themselves to notice how you look!! Wear a towel or full bodied suit, but get your hiney in that pool!!".

Here is a timeline of the changes and experiences you can expect to go through. If you don't experience your body change in accordance with my time frame, it's ok. People's bodies are different! However, if you don't make huge progress within 4-5 months, you are doing something wrong; chances are it's your eating and/or you're not prioritizing you're not making time for your workouts.

Android Timeline

Month		
	1	Uuuck!! This hurts I don't think I like this!
	2	But strangely, I am starting to feel things that were never there before....-muscles???
	3	Ok, I can see this is really starting to work, and you know, I don't feel as bad as I did before!
	4	Alright. I'm addicted to this, sign me up!
	5	Arg! I seem to have been hitting this plateau for about 2-3 weeks, I need help!
	6	Doing better, losing weight but very small amounts, 1/2 pound- 1 lb every 2 weeks or so.
	7	Wow, that just kind of snuck up on me! I am 2/3rds the way to my goal!

Christin H. McDowell

Progressive Training Programs for the Androidian Woman

You are a Beginner if...

- you have been inactive or not working out for more than 6 months
- you're at low risk (initial assessment Chapter 2)
- you just want to start off easy

Programs include 7 day Layouts and training routines for Weight Training, Track and Pool. Track and Pool Workouts start on page 120.

1. Months 1-3   **Beginner**
2. Months 4-6   **Intermediate**
3. Months 7+   **Advanced**

CV: Your cardio needs to stay within either your THRZ (Target Heart Rate Zone) or your HRR (Heart Rate Reserve). You should have calculated this out, if not, grab a calculator and do it! It will be important for you to stick within that range if you're just starting out, or if you have risk factors (Chapter 2). In the beginning, it's important to keep your heart rate at a steady beat and MINIMIZE intervals. This is because you don't want to shock your system when first starting out. Allow your heart and lungs plenty of time to strengthen and get healthier.

LT CV: Light Cardio: Go Easy.

Some options for Cardio:

- Walking outside
- Elliptical- try to use one that involves your arms
- Treadmill
- Stair Stepper, Stepmill
- Versa Climber
- Minimize the bike unless you are tired (because you're sitting down and moving only ½ your body)
- Walking Hand Weights
- Pool

Walking Hand Weights are a great way to burn fat and build muscle tone. You can use hand weights on a walkway, gym, on a track or even in your home!

Good Hand Weight Exercises: (See Exercise Reference section)

1. Curl Turn Press Bi2
2. Back Row (like a lawn mower) B8
3. Walking Triceps Extension Tri2
4. Upper Cuts, Punches S6, S7

You want to do each arm exercise until it starts burning a bit, then switch to the next exercise. You can do one arm at a time or both. A good rep range is 6-15 each arm, using 2-6lbs dumbbells. Take a break after you have done one round, set the weights down, walk regularly, and then pick them up again for Round 2!

Shoot for 3-5 Rounds or 10-15 min.

7 Day Layout and Workout

Monday	Tuesday	Wednesday	Thursday	Friday	Saturday	Sunday
CV 40Min WRKT 1	LT CV 35-50min CR OR POOL 1/2	OFF	CV 45 Min OR Pool Weights	CV 45 CR 5 OR POOL 1/2	PA/OFF	OFF

Exercise	Sets	Reps	Weight	Reference #
Push Ups	2-3	8-10 or	BDWT	C2
on Knees or feet		10-15		
Back Row	2-3	8 to 15	MOD	B4
Dumbell or Barbell				B1
Plank Hold on hands	2-3	15-30	BDWT	CR8
		sec		
Triceps Dips	2-3	8 to 12	BDWT	Tri3
		or 10-20		
Alternate Biceps Curl	2-3	6 to 15	LT-MOD	PB2
(Not on Physioball)				
Basic Crunch	2-3	10-15	BDWT or	CR1
or Barbell Crunch			45LBS which	
JHRT!!	2-3	1 MIN 20s		J 1-4
		total		
Walking Step Up	2-3	8-10	BDWT or hold	L17
			8lb dmbls	
Pickers	2-3	6-10	BDWT or hold	L10 or L11
			8lb dmbls	
Elliptical or Treadmill	2-3	2-4 MIN		

Months 4-6: Intermediate

7 Day Layout and Workout

Monday	Tuesday	Wednesday	Thursday	Friday	Saturday	Sunday
Warm Up 5-10min Workout 1	CV 60min Land or Pool	OFF Or 60min CV	Warm Up 5-10min Workout 1	CV 60min Land or Pool	PA 45-1HR	OFF

Exercise	Sets	Reps	Weight		Reference #
Push Ups	2	8-10	BDWT		C2
Mtn Climbers	2	15-20	MOD		J4
Up Up/Down Downs	2	5 Each Arm	BDWT	Stage 1	CR10
Full sit up		20sec			CR5
Back Row Barbell	2	15	45lbs		B1
Triceps Dips	2	or 10-20	BDWT		Tri3
JHR!!		6 to 15			J 1-4
45° Chest Press	2-3	10-15	45LBS+		C1
DMBL Back Row	2-3	12-15	12-20 lbs		B4
Narrow Lat Pull	2	8-10	Mod		B5
ss. Wide Lat Pull	2	8-12	LT	Stage 2	B6
Squat Curl Turn Press SS	2	8	6+lb Dumbells		L13,S3
JHR, Elliptical 45-1m Sprint	2-3		Intense		J 1-4
Pickers	2	6-8	BDWT or 6+ Dumbells		L10 or L11
Step Ups	2	6-8	(Same)	Stage 3	L17
Stair Stepper Sprint 45s	2	2-4 MIN			
Finish With Core Work					CR-

7 Day Layout and Workout

Monday	Tuesday	Wednesday	Thursday	Friday	Saturday	Sunday
WTS 40 Min CV: 20 min	CV 60min POOL or Track Workout	OFF	WTS CV: 20 min	CV 60min POOL Or Track Workout	LT CV 45-60min	OFF or PA

Exercise	Sets	Reps	Weight		Reference #
Run Warm Up 800M				Stage 1	
Med Ball Plyos:	2		6-8lb Medball		M
Medball Chest Pass	2	10-15	MOD		M1
Medball Toss Up	2	20meters	BDWT		M2
Medball Triceps Ext.	2	20			M3
High Knee Skips	2	20meters			J1
Sprints	3-5+	about 30-			
		50m+			
Push Up Pops	2	10-15	BDWT	Stage 2	C10
Back Row Pops	2	10-20	BDWT		B1
Up/Up Down Down's	2	5-8	BDWT		CR10
Mtn Climbers	2	15-25	BDWT		J4
Band Press on Bosu	2	15-20	Red or Blue Band		C13
45° Chest Press	2	10-15	45LBS+		C1
Bosu Double Arm Band Back Row	2	10-20	Red or Blue Band		BB2
DMBL Back Row	2	12-15	12-20 lbs		B4

Elliptical Sprints 2min					
JHR					J 1-4
Plie Hops	2	10-15	BDWT or Wtd		L12
Stationary Lung Hop	2	8-10	BDWT or Wtd		L16
or Double Leg Hop	2	10-15	BDWT or Wtd	**Stage 3**	L19
Step Ups Alternate (Opt. Fast)	2	6-8	BDWT or Wtd		L17
400m Run	2	6-8			
Full sit Up to Jumps	2	6-8		**Stage 4**	CR12
Press, Crunch, Butt Lifts	2	2-4 MIN	25-45lbs		CR11
Finish With Core Work			3-5min		CR-

Gynoid Women

Gynoid body fat is pear-shaped in hip and thigh

Being 'Gynoid' presents us with unique challenges over our Androidian friends. They can parade around in their bathing suits carrying around an extra 10-30lbs without a hint of cellulite. We Gynoiders on the other hand, show every additional *ounce* of fat on our butts and thighs. Ours is a tough challenge but that doesn't mean that we're not up to the task! We can all make the best of our bodies; our mission is to do it!

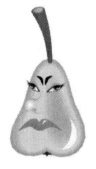

So what is a Gynoider and what does she look like?

Honestly... **somewhat like a juicy pear**... big butt, big hips, smaller waist, either small or medium arms, but definitely got the large booty. She may have a hard time getting to her desired jean size, but I can assure you, doing these workouts and eating like a 'Healthy Tart', will ensure success.

The Pro's

1. You will probably live longer than an androider because the bulk of your fat is located away from your organs. From a health standpoint, it's better to have excess fat on your butt than on your belly.
2. With the proper training, your upper body will change very fast.
3. With training, your butt will end up being the envy of those Androidians!

The Con's

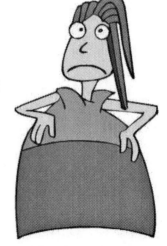

1. You will have to adopt a new (unyielding) healthy eating regime to keep off the cellulite and get rid of the big butt. Everything you need to know about healthy eating can be found in 'Healthy Tart'.
2. Your lower body fat will be the last to go!

Your Training Recommendations

1. No real heavy weight training, unless you want to gain bulk.
2. High Reps, light weight for your upper body.
3. You will need to Super set exercises to make sure your heart rate is up.
4. You will need to embrace the thing you hate the most, i.e. running. Your body will change fast as a result.
5. Cardio, cardio, cardio. And...change it up. E.g., if all you do is 60 min on the elliptical, that ain't changing it up!
6. Lay off lifting heavy weights for your legs; they will respond better with body weight exercises, running and swimming. If you can't run or swim, work up to it. YOU CAN eventually, believe in yourself. You can also do sprints on the cardio machines.
7. Cleanse out your intestines; you probably won't see the cellulite go until you do! Chances are there are extra toxins around your glutes and thighs because of the toxic build up in your organs. Refer to the '30 Day Detox' in 'Healthy Tart'.
8. You will lose a substantial amount of size in your upper body during the first 1-3 months; if you're doing everything right...after which you may well hit a plateau before your legs start changing. Just double your determination for eating right and pick the intensity up for your workouts.
9. Use Pool workouts to help elongate your body and give it a good workout. All the pool workouts start on page 123. Choose which best suits you; it doesn't matter if you can't swim, I have workouts for all levels and abilities!

So my fellow Gynoiders; you will have to be very smart about the way you eat and train but just remember, if you follow the program and (most importantly) hit up the cardio, it's gonna happen! You WILL get to your goals. SO STICK WITH IT!

For more information and resources, go to www.TrishaStewart.com, www.ChristinMcDowell.com or watch my training DVD's for further guidance.

Gynoid Timeline

Month	1	Uuuck!! This hurts I don't think I like this!
	2	Wow, I've lost a couple of inches in my upper body already!
	3	My upper body is definitely changing but my legs and butt are staying the same!
	4	Ok, will I have these saddle bags for LIFE?
	5	Alright, I'm finally seeing results with my lower body...
	6	Hit a plateau on the scale, but I know I can do better with my eating
	7	Wow, that just kind of snuck up on me! I am 2/3rds the way to my goal!

You are a Beginner if...

- you have been inactive or not working out for more than 6 months
- you're at low risk (initial assessment Chapter 2)
- you just want to start off easy

Programs include 7 day Layouts and training routines for Weight Training, Track and Pool

4. **Months 1-3**   **Beginner**
5. **Months 4-6**   **Intermediate**
6. **Months 7+**   **Advanced**

CV: Your cardio needs to stay within either your THRZ (Target Heart Rate Zone) or your HRR (Heart Rate Reserve). You should have calculated this out, if not, grab a calculator and do it! It will be important for you to stick within that range if you're just starting out, or if you have risk factors (Chapter 2). In the beginning, it's important to keep your heart rate at a steady beat and MINIMIZE intervals. This is because you don't want to shock your system when first starting out. Allow your heart and lungs plenty of time to strengthen and get healthier.

LT CV: Light Cardio, Go Easy

Some options for Cardio:

- Walking outside
- Elliptical- try to use one that involves your arms
- Treadmill
- Stair Stepper, Step mill
- Versa Climber

- Minimize the bike unless you are tired (because you're sitting down and moving only ½ your body)
- Walking Hand Weights

Stirring up the Cardio Options!

It's really important you constantly change up and progress your cardio intensity and variety. Here are some examples:

Treadmill:

- Run a short distance then walk... try to hit goals either with time or distance, e.g. time: 2 min run or on a treadmill .25 of a mile, which is 400meters. Then try to do it at a faster pace and more often
- Adding a 2-3% incline during your recovery increases intensity and really blasts fat! Outdoor running programs are included

Elliptical/Crosstrainer Machine:

1. Push/Pull: focus on pushing forwards with your arms or backwards to accent different muscle groups
2. Sprints: put it on a harder, higher level and going fast for time, e.g. going medium pace at level 7, sprinting at level 10 for 20 sec.
3. Go Backwards: keep your hips back to accent your glutes and hamstrings
4. Hard/Easy: choose a comfortable intensity then bump it up to a very hard level, and just keep it moving for a certain amount of time. eg. easy at level 7, hard at level 15 for 20 sec., then recovering again at level 7

I have provided **Track and Pool** workouts that are included in your programs. Refer to page 120.

7 Day Layout and Workout

Monday	Tuesday	Wednesday	Thursday	Friday	Saturday	Sunday
CV 40Min WRKT 1	CV 35-50min OR POOL	LT CV 40Min OR OFF	POOL	WRKT 1	45-60Min CV	OFF

Exercise	Sets	Reps	Weight		Reference #
Push Ups (Knees, Feet)	2	6-8	BDWT		
Basic Crunch	2	8-12	BDWT		CR1
Plank Hold on hands	2	30s	BDWT		CR8
Triceps Dips	2	10	BDWT		Tri3
Barbell Row	2	8-12	BDWT		B1
Single Arm Row	2	8 to 12	8-12LBS	Stage 1	B4
Band Biceps Curl	2	or 10-20	Mod		Bi1
2 min Elliptical	2		Intense!		
JHRT!!					J 1-4
Plie	2	8-10	BDWT or		L13
Pickers	2	8-12	BDWT or 8lbs		L10, L11
Abduction	2	1 MIN 20s	Mod		L1
JHRT!!	2				J 1-4
Step Up	2	6-8 Each leg	BDWT		L17
Stair Stepper	2	20-30 Sec	BDWT or hold	Stage 2	
Walk or Run	1	3-5 Min	Mod-Int		
Stretch		2-4 MIN			

Months 4-6: Intermediate

---

7 Day Layout and Workout

Monday	Tuesday	Wednesday	Thursday	Friday	Saturday	Sunday
CV 60Min Land	WRKT 1	CV 60Min Pool	OFF	CV 60min Land or Pool	Choose Any Wts 25min CV 45min	OFF

Exercise	Sets	Reps	Weight		Reference #
Warm Up 5-10min	1				
Plies	2	10-15	BDWT		L13
Step Ups	2	6 Each Leg	BDWT		L17
JHRT!!	2				J 1-4
Push Ups	2	10-15	BDWT	Stage 1	C2
Barbell Back Rows	2	10-20	Barbell 45lbs		B1
Up Up/Down Downs	2	5 Each Arm	BDWT		CR10
JHRT!!	2				J 1-4
2 min Ellip	2				
Wide Leg Press	2	15-20	BDWT or LT		L18
Narrow Leg Press	2	15-20	BDWT or LT	Stage 2	L9
Walking Luge	2	6 Each leg	BDWT or LT		L7
JHRT!!	2				J 1-4
Physioball Crunch	2	15	BDWT		CR6
Physioball Plank Hold	2	20-30Sec	BDWT		CR7
Wide Grip Lat Pull Away	2	8-10	LT	Stage 3	B6
Narrow Grip Lat Pull Face	2	6-8	MOD		B5

Christin H. McDowell

Stair Stepper	2	30Sec	Intense!		
Elliptical Sprint	1	45Sec-1min	Intense!		
Band Chest Press	1	10-20	LT AND FAST!		C3
Band Back Row	1	15-20	LT AND FAST!		B2
Band Curls	1	10-15	LT AND FAST!		Bi1
Triceps Body Weight Dips	1	10-15	BDWT	Stage 4	Tri3
2 Min Ellip	1	2 MIN	MOD		
CORE		5 MIN			CR-

Months 7+: Advanced

---

7 Day Layout and Workout

Monday	Tuesday	Wednesday	Thursday	Friday	Saturday	Sunday
Workout 1 CV: 20 min Sprints	CV 60min POOL or Track Workout	OFF Or Pool	60 Min CV	Choose Rx's From WRKT 1	LT CV 60min	OFF or PA

Exercise	Sets	Reps	Weight		Reference #
Sprints:					
5x 20m	1				
High knee Skips	2	20Meters			J1
Medball Chest Pass	2	10-15	6-8lb Medball	Stage 1	M1
Double leg jumps	2	15-20 Jumps			L19
Run 50-100m	1				
JHRT!!	1				J 1-4
2 min Elliptical Sprint	1				
Plie Hops	2	12-15	BDWT		L12
Stationary Lunge Hop or alt.	2	10	BDWT		L16
Step up or Step up Hops	2	6-10	BDWT	Stage 2	L17
Barbell Back Row	2	15-20	BDWT		B1
Push Up Pops	2	10-20	BDWT		C10
Full Sit Up to Jumps	2	8-10	BDWT		CR12
Wide Grip Lat Pull Face	1-2	6-8	MOD		B5
Narrow Grip Lat Pull Away	1-2	8-12	LT		B6
Back Row Bands	2	15-25	LT AND FAST	Stage 3	B2
Band Chest Press	2	10-15	LT AND FAST		C3

Band Curls	2	6-12	LT AND FAST		Bi1
Up/Up Down Downs	2	5-6 Each	BDWT		CR10
Triceps Body Weight Dips	2	12-20	BDWT		Tri3
Sprints:					
Elliptical	3	30-45Sec	Back to Back		
Stair Stepper	3	25-40Sec	if Possible	Stage 4	
Bike Sprints	2-3	20-30Sec off,			
		15 Sec on			
Finish with 2 min Cool Down					
Core		5 Min			CR

*Go as quick as you can from one thing to the next, with little or no rest time.

Women United

"The definition of insanity is doing the same thing over and over and expecting different results." Benjamin Franklin

If you want to avoid gaining a whole bunch of bulky muscle, but really want to lose body fat, you must be smart and varied with your workouts. Cardio workouts should be interesting and fun! You want to burn fat and tighten your body so:

- Run
- Swim
- Hike
- Dance
- Jump
- Cycle
- Climb

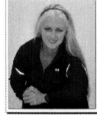

Christin's Tip!

Re-educate your body! If you love weights but hate running; run more. If you like the elliptical but hate the stair stepper; do the stair stepper! If you enjoying swimming but always do breaststroke, mix it up with backstroke and the crawl. Never be monotonous in your workouts! Shocking your body will burn a ton of calories and rapidly increase your fitness!

Take a good multivitamin, and extra antioxidants with your new program. Your body will need more vitamins and minerals to repair tissue damage and replenish stores. You'll spare yourself injury, burnout, have more energy and feel better.

Take rest days! Rest days are necessary in order for your body to recover from intense exercise. Don't fall into the trap of over training or over extending your body early in your training program.

But just as important... don't convince yourself that you need to rest your body when all you really want is to avoid working out! In other words, DON'T BE LAZY! Your body will let you know when it needs rest; you'll know the difference.

Try to work out with a friend or in a group; it's much more motivational when you get a friendly rivalry going. You'll be more inclined to go for that run if you have company or are just trying to compete with your neighbor. Bottom line: do whatever it takes to stay on track and keep motivated!

Chapter 6

Stability and Balance Training

"Without balance at all times, you can never be effective"
Bruce Lee

The Central Nervous System (CNS) is engaged in everything we do; both consciously and unconsciously. It is the network that transports messages from your brain to every part of your body and it is the system that controls balance and stability.

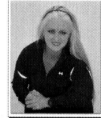

Christin's Tip!

Specific stability and balance training is totally unimportant when you're first starting out compared to getting deadly weight off and improving the condition of your heart and lungs. The CNS is active in everything you do, so even something as simple as walking helps with stability.

The Stability and Balance exercises that follow are to be incorporated into your total fitness program when you have reached your target weight. Don't waste your time and effort until your body itself is in balance!

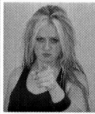

Christin's Rant!

I hate it when I see trainers putting their severely overweight clients on a 'Bosu ball' when they have not a drop of sweat or even a hint of a flushed face. It's unacceptable to me.
What's the good of doing funky moves on a Bosu if you're going to have a heart attack soon? GET THE WEIGHT OFF FIRST, then worry about becoming an acrobatic ninja!!

Stability Training and its importance for the Elderly

Unlike their younger counterparts, balance and stability training is vitally important for the elderly. A significant cause of death in the elderly is a suppressed immune system; brought on by a bone fracture (usually caused by a fall). When a bone breaks, the immune system has to work overtime to heal the damaged site, but it can only cope with so much. Pneumonia and other sicknesses can be deadly to a weakened immune system.

Balance and stability training help prevent those falls from ever happening!

Stability training and its importance for Athletes

For athletic performance, balance and stability can be the difference between winning and losing games! The ability of a wide receiver to catch a ball four feet up in the air, land on one foot, stay inbounds and then sprint towards the end zone is an example of generating power through active stability training.

Like all exercise 'tactics', specific stability and balance training has its place when the time and conditions are right.

Stability and Balance Exercises

<u>Physioball Dumbell Chest Press</u>

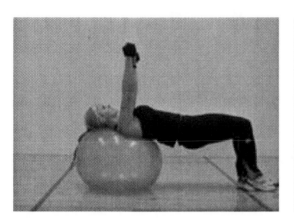 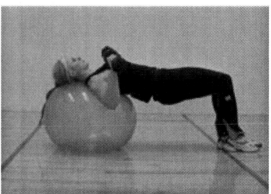

- Keep your feet and knees together
- Lift your butt up high and keep it tight
- Place your hands so the thumbs face each other
- Keep your head on the ball

- Lower arms down so your elbows are at 90°
- Keep arms at 45°
- Keep shoulders down
- Squeeze your abs and exhale as you Press back up

Physioball Dumbell Chest Fly

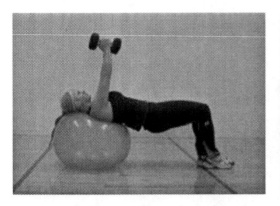 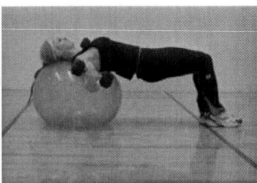

- Keep your feet and knees together
- Lift your butt up high and keep it tight
- Place your hands so they are facing each other
- Keep your head on the ball

- Reach out to the sides with your Arms
- Keep a slight bend in your Arms
- Pretend like you are give a bear hug to someone
- Keep your shoulders down as your bring your hands back together

Physioball Dumbell Pullover

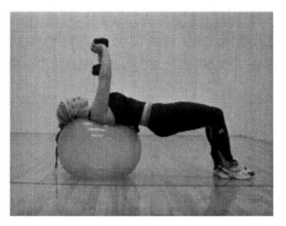 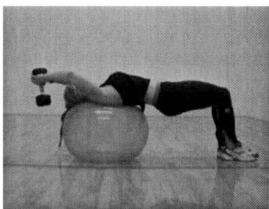

- Keep your feet and knees together
- Lie on the ball, so your Head is fully on the ball
- Make a triangle with your hands
- Hold the dumbell over your Chest

- Reach back with your arms
- Keep a slight bend in arms
- Pull back to start position using Lats

Physioball Plank Hold/and or Roll

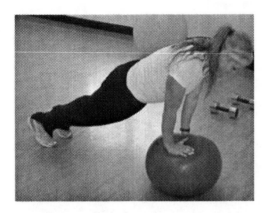

- Keep hands directly underneath your chest on the ball
- Keep your back straight
- Keep your butt down

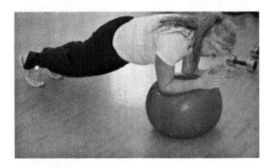

- Gently roll down onto your elbows maintaining a tight back and waist
- Keep hands straight forward

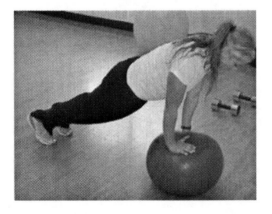

- Exhale as you use your arm and shoulder strength to move yourself back up to the start position
- Keep your butt down

Physioball Crunch

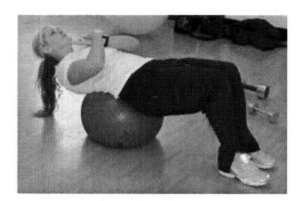 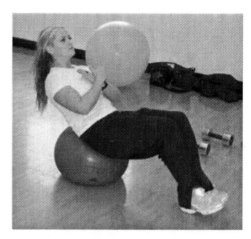

- Keep knees together
- Keep feet together
- Keep Back slightly bent back-Abdominal wall fully extended
- Stabilize the ball before any movement
- Inhale
- Hands cross the chest or supporting the neck

- Keep back straight as you lift
- Stop right before you have no more tension

Physioball Biceps Curl

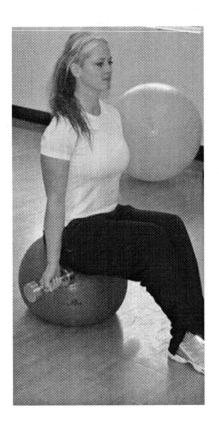 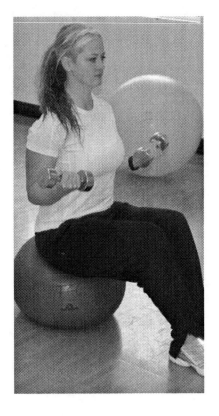

- Keep knees together
- Keep feet together
- Keep arms fully extended
- Chest out
- Shoulders back
- Stabilize the ball before any movement
- Inhale

- Curl and exhale
- Arms go straight up, keeping hands straight up
- Keeping knees and feet TOGETHER

Physioball Dumbell Shoulder Raise

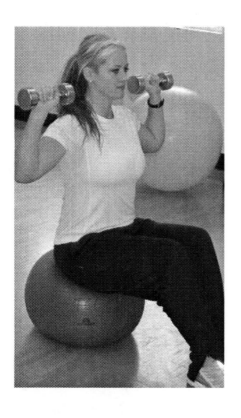 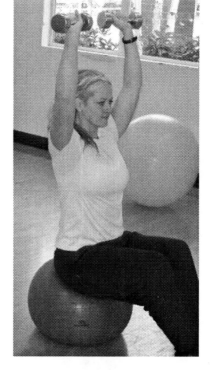

- Keep knees together
- Keep feet together
- Keep hands at 90°
- Chest out
- Shoulders back
- Stabilize the ball before any movement

- Press and exhale
- Fully extend at your arms
- Keeping knees and feet TOGETHER
- Go straight up not forward

Bosu Bands Chest Press

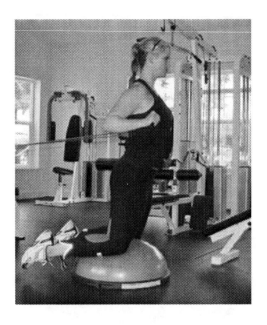 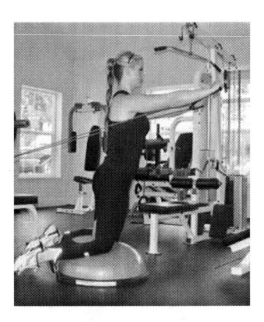

- Chest Out
- Shoulders Back
- Elbows at 45°
- Both knees on Bosu, hip width apart
- Use your chest not your shoulders
- Keep Core Tight! You can have the band at an angle as an Incline Chest Press, or you can have it level, as a Flat Chest Press

- Keep your Feet off the ground
- Fully extend your arms
- Slightly lean into the motion
- You can Do Single Arms or Doubles
- Still stay tight

Bosu Band Back Row

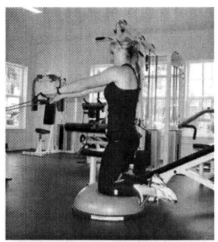

- Chest Out
- Extend shoulders out
- Both knees hip width apart on the bosu
- Start with your hands facing down
- Keep Core Tight

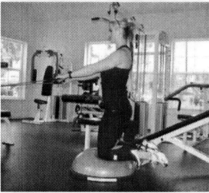

- Retract...
- Don't drop your head down

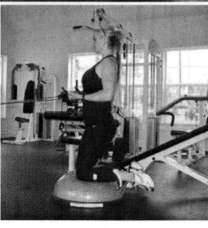

- Turn and pull
- Keep shoulders down, chest out
- You can Do Single Arms or Doubles
- Squeeze below your shoulder blades, this is where you should feel it.

Bosu Ab Hold

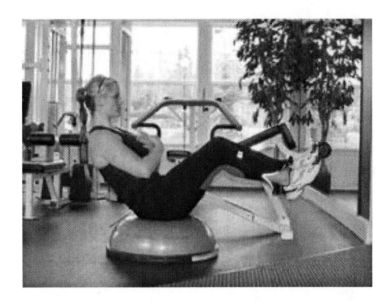

- Sit in the middle of the Bosu
- Lean back slightly
- Keep your knees up and Hold

Bosu Plank Hold

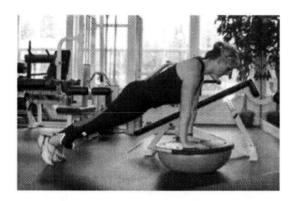 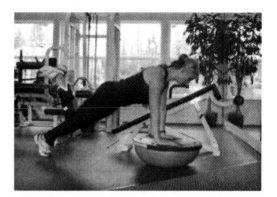

- Place your hands shoulder width apart on the Bosu, face them forward
- Get in a Plank Hold position
- Stay on the balls of your Feet
- Keep your butt down, don't sag your Lower Back

- You can make this exercise harder by lifting up 1 Leg, Moving your Arms side to side or forward and backwards

<u>Bosu Squat</u>

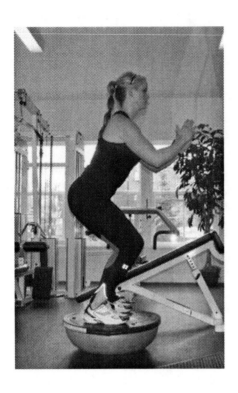 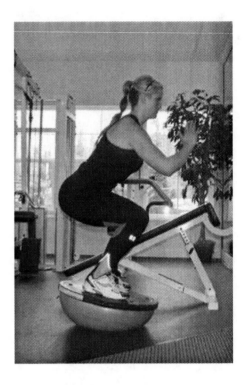

- Keep feet hip width apart
- Slight bend in knees
- Keep hips back
- Chest out, shoulders back, stay retracted
- Stay in the Middle of the Bosu
- You can put 1 foot on and then step onto the Bosu, or you can jump onto it

- As you keep your hips back, lower down to 90°
- Keep Back straight
- As you stand back up, focus on having stability-little movement
- You can make this harder by moving your legs side to side or forwards and backwards-staying down

Chapter 7

Stretching

"I do some weights and I do a lot of stretching."
Mike Ditka

Stretching promotes an increased range of motion and can prevent injury. Stretching relaxes over tight muscles and helps with muscular imbalances (see chapter 2).

If a muscle feels tight, stretch for 10-45 seconds, or until it starts to relax. Stretch a muscle when it's warm; if you don't, it's like taking a rubber band, sticking in the freezer and pulling on it: the result; it snaps. So warm up and workout, but if you feel tightness, stretch.

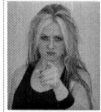

Christin's Rant!
When you workout, WORKout!

I see too many overweight people come to the gym and sit down to stretch for the majority of their workout. They come and go and their bodies never change. I wonder why...!

If you have areas that always seem tight, don't further stress them with weight training. The muscle is letting you know it's being overused and needs a break. Get a massage and gently stretch it out.

Movement promotes range of motion, circulation and flexibility. If you're tight, get in the pool and gently aqua jog or swim.

Foam rollers are an effective tool for overactive muscle tissue. They help loosen tight muscles and increase circulation. You can hold the foam roller on the tight muscle, or roll it

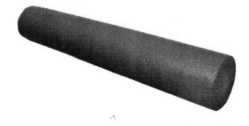

over back and forth. Hold it as long as you need until you feel the muscle tissue start to relax.

Stretching and Athletic Performance:

Stretching increases range of motion which will help the potential for power production. It's important not to overstretch as it will lead to a decrease of potential force/power. Hold the stretch until you feel like the muscle is ready; anywhere from 10-30 seconds. Working on stretching out your muscular imbalances is very important, as well as promoting flexibility in your groin and hamstrings (injury prone areas). For muscle groups that are constantly tense, try to lay off of them, get massages and stretch.

<u>Glute Stretches</u>

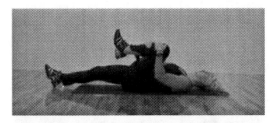

- Lie on back
- Pull knee to chest
- Keep opposite leg straight

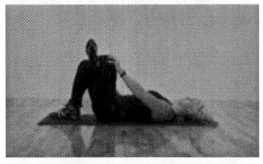

- Cross leg over
- Keep legs bent
- Press knee down gently

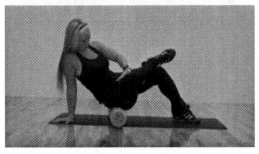

- Use a foam roll for added stretch release
- Press knee down if necessary

Groin

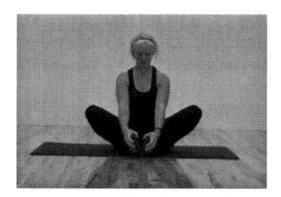 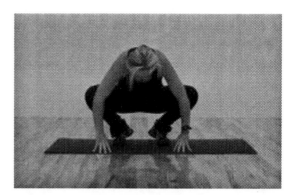

- Sit
- Place feet together, work legs down
- You can press down on your knees for an added pull

- Can also be done squatting
- Press your knees out with your arms
- Gently lean into the stretch

Lower Back

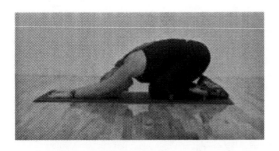

- Reach arms forward
- Sit Butt to heels
- Round and straighten spine

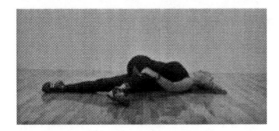

- Reach your leg across your body
- Keep your opposite shoulder down (my right shoulder)

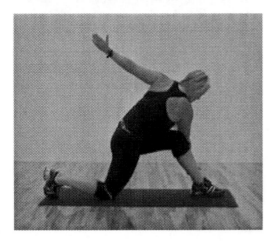

- Get in a hip flexor stretch
- Turn your torso so your opposite elbow is behind your lead leg
- You can also reach your arm out to make it more advanced

<u>Hamstring</u>

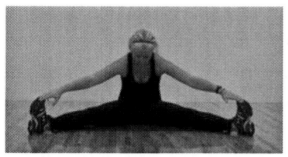 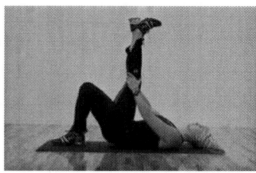

- Spread legs
- Reach forward to toes
- Keep back straight

- Extend leg up and pull back

<u>Quadriceps</u>

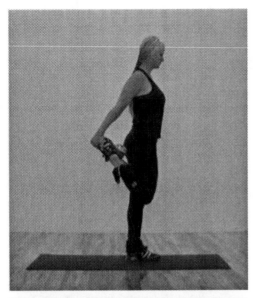

- Keep both feet straight
- Pull up on foot until you feel a comfortable pull in your quadriceps (front of your thigh)

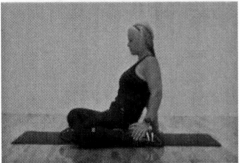

- You can also sit down and fold your legs
- Make sure to keep both legs bent

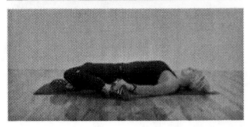

- Or lying down as well

Upper Body Stretches

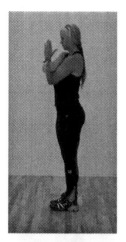

- Posterior Deltoid:
- Keep both feet straight
- Bring arm across Body and hold
- Thumb stays up)

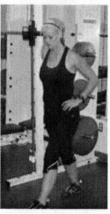

- Chest Stretch:
- Open Chest up as you hold arm to wall
- Slightly turn body

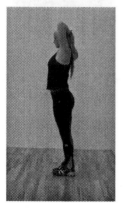

- Lat and Shoulder:
- Pull arm behind head
- Slightly lean upper body in direction of the pull OR
- Lean up against wall and sink hips back as you pull with arms

Foam Roll Examples

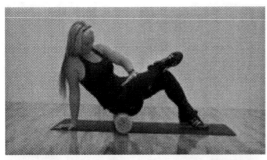

- Glute

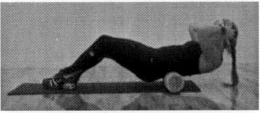

- Lower Back

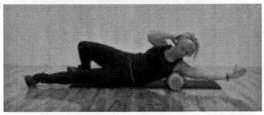

- Lat

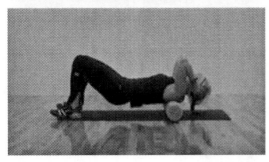

- Upper Back

Chapter 8

Pregnancy and Fitness

"The breasts go first, and then the waist and then the butt. Nobody ever tells you that you get a butt when you get pregnant." Elle Macpherson

If you're considering having a child, your personal health and fitness is crucial to the health of both you and your baby; both during and after pregnancy... so do your best to get in shape and adopt a healthy lifestyle before you conceive! I recommend a copy of 'Healthy Tart' and 'Healthy Idol' for advice on nutrition and lifestyle issues.

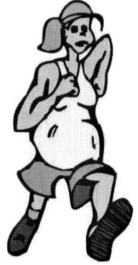

My Gynoid and Android workouts cover everything you need to get in shape; before you conceive... so revisit them and come back here when you're pregnant!

If you are pregnant, it's important you start slowly and be comfortable with the exercises you do. I have provided some light exercises which will help support and strengthen your body during pregnancy.

Benefits of Exercise for the Pregnant Mother and Baby

❖ Increased circulation nutrients and oxygen to the growing fetus and mother
❖ When you exercise, endorphins (happy hormones) are released; which will stimulate both you and the baby making for a happier, healthier pregnancy
❖ Exercise helps prevent gestational diabetes
❖ It can reduce the risk of birth defects
❖ It can reduce pre and post natal depression
❖ Lower Risk of delivering asphyxiated babies (babies that don't have enough oxygen)
❖ You'll be able to lose the weight quicker after birth
❖ A healthier and stronger placenta
❖ A stronger immune system
❖ Can enhance development of baby's cerebral cortex
❖ Can lead to easier birthing
❖ Newborns tend to be more alert and calm
❖ Helps improve maternal mental functioning
❖ Helps reduce stress

Exercise Tips

- ❖ Stay Hydrated! Dehydration during exercise can cause premature labor
- ❖ Don't get too hot or too cold; maintain a consistent and comfortable environment
- ❖ Take adequate time to warm up and cool down, 10+ minutes
- ❖ Don't overstretch. Your hormones are enabling your joints to be extra flexible, so it will be easier to pull a muscle or overextend it. Contrary to what you might have heard, yoga can be risky during pregnancy
- ❖ Your workouts shouldn't be intense; it's better to have longer easier workouts depending. Don't work to the point of 'shortness of breath' and don't hold your breath during exercise

Check with your doctor to make sure you're healthy enough to exercise; especially during pregnancy.

If you don't already exercise regularly...
You really shouldn't start a new (intense) exercise program. Just stick to walking or light swimming.

If you <u>do</u> already exercise regularly...
In the beginning you don't really need to change anything, just don't raise your internal temperature too much and don't lift heavy weights. As you're your baby continues to develop, there are some adjustments you need to make with your workouts. Always discuss what you are doing with your doctor.

Trimester Tips and Tools

Your body will change through each trimester so you will need to adjust your workouts accordingly.

Trimester 1:

Gently start strengthening your abdomen, your upper and lower back. They need to be strong to support the added weight you will be carrying around; especially during trimester 3:

Exercises:

1. Single Arm Back Row –OR
   do any or all of the back exercises: B
2. Band Back Rows –B2
3. Band Chest Press –C3
4. Triceps Dips –Tri3
5. Incline Chest Press –C4

6. Basic Crunch -CR1
7. Side Crunches -CR9
8. Seated Curl turn Press -Bi2
9. Deltoid Raises -S1
10. Gentle Supermen, or a lower back machine that can be accessed in the gym
11. Walking hand weights:

    a. Walking Curl Turn Press -Bi2
    b. Triceps Extension -Tri2
    c. Walking Punch -S6
    d. Upper Cut -S7

Make sure the reps are higher-12-15 and that you are breathing through the range of motion. Use light to moderate weight, never heavy weights. 2 Sets would be fine. Make sure your breathing is regulated so that you get plenty of oxygen.

Trimester 2:

- Most doctors recommend that pregnant women avoid exercises after the first trimester that requires them to lie flat on their backs
- Don't get out of breath, make sure you can breathe the whole time; again, it's better to go easier for a longer time then harder for a shorter amount of time

Trimester 3:

- Pool, Pool, Pool! This will enable you to relax, stretch your body out and vent out some energy from feeling so restricted with carrying around excess weight
- I'm not comfortable with the idea of pregnant women in their 3rd trimester doing yoga because of the hyper-mobility of their joints especially as they get closer to the birth their baby

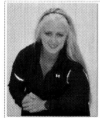

Christin's Tip!

It is often the pregnant mother who can best determine what intensity and duration she is able to do because of her past exercise history and being in tune with her body

STOP exercising if you experience:

- Sudden and severe abdominal pain
- Uterine contractions lasting 30 minutes once exercise stops
- Decreased fetal activity
- Dizziness and vaginal bleeding
- Visual problems
- Numbness in any part of the body
- Overheating

Fortunately, after the birth of your beautiful new baby, losing the weight should be easier if you have stayed active and healthy during your pregnancy... so relax, be patient and start things off slow. Easy does it at first, then step-up the intensity and duration of your exercise. You can start off again as a beginner Androidian or Gynoider, or intermediate etc., (chapter 4)!

Chapter 9

MYTHS, Q & A!

"There'll always be some weird thing about eating four grapes before you go to bed, or drinking a special tea, or buying this little bean from El Salvador." Richard Simmons

Myth #1: If I do a whole bunch of sit-ups my gut will go away

No matter how many crunches and sit ups you do, it WON'T make your gut go away unless you burn the fat that's in it! Losing your belly is about burning total calories and eating well. How many calories do you think you are burning by doing 15 min of crunches vs. 15 min of sprints? You can't even compare the two!

Myth #2: Working out 2-3x/wk is good enough for <u>weight loss</u>

Not so. The recommendation for WEIGHT LOSS is 1 HR OF CARDIO MOST DAYS OF THE WEEK. That's right; 1 HR of solid cardio most days of the week. Typically it'll be men who tell you that you don't need to do more cardio because they have much more lean muscle tissue and better hormones for burning calories and body fat. However, if you are female like me, and it is quite easy to get fat in a matter of days, 3x/wk is not going to cut it. (See page 60 for a full explanation)

#3: If I just eat less and workout more I'll lose weight; I can do it on my own!

IF YOU HAVE BEEN TALKING ABOUT EXERCISE FOR MORE THAN A YEAR, 6 MONTHS, OR EVEN 3 WEEKS, AND YOU STILL ARE NOT EXERCISING <u>REGULARLY,</u> (3-6x's/wk) YOU HAVE PROVED TO YOURSELF THAT YOU NEED HELP. And that's OK!!! This book along with 'Healthy Tart' for women, 'Healthy Dude Book' for men, provides everything you need to get in shape; if you put in the effort. Trisha Stewart's website, www.trishastewart.com, is an online resource for accountability, support, as well as a full set of physical training videos; so I can be YOUR virtual trainer!

#4: Lifting weights or doing body weight exercises makes women develop big muscles.

Wrong. It takes a lot of time, energy and focus to get your muscles bigger.

1. First, if you are on a restricted caloric diet, which many people are, it will be virtually impossible for your muscles to grow much bigger. The key is how you train, what you eat and even how much cardio you're doing.
2. Testosterone, and other male dominant hormones, boosts the development of muscle tissue. That's why men respond so much more rapidly to weight training than women. So have no fear girls, unless you're relatively short and are a genetic magnet, you'll have a hard time gaining a whole bunch of muscle mass.

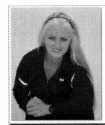

Christin's Tip!

If you're a woman and your goal is weight, don't be so sore you can't move the next day; as you won't be able to burn any more calories and further your fitness.

Question #1: How do I get rid of my gut?

By reducing your total body fat. Your body draws and stores fat wherever it wants to. The big idea is to BURN total body fat. How many calories do you think you're burning from doing 5 min of crunches? Hardly any. Abdominal exercises merely strengthen your muscles, not burn a whole bunch of fat. Exercise to burn calories, and that gut, along with eating well, will go away.

Question #2: How do I get rid of my Saddle Bags (sagging thighs)?

Again, a simple reduction of total body fat! See above!

You can strengthen and support the muscle tissue in those areas to add shape, but ultimately, workout to burn fat!

Here are some exercises to help you shape up your figure in your lower body. Use the Exercise Reference Section for reference to these exercises. Remember, cardio will kick your butt in shape FAST, so focus on manipulating the mode!

- Good Cardio Choices: Running, Bleachers, Stair stepper, Ellipticals, Versa Climber
- Weight Training and body weight exercises: 2-3 sets, 15-25 reps

  a. Plies
  b. Lunges
  c. Step ups
  d. Squats
  e. Leg press
  f. Machines: Inner/Outer Thigh, Quad Extensions, Hamstring Curls
  g. Iso (Self Contracted): Adduction/Abduction, Bent leg kick, straight leg kick

Question #3: How can I lose my bat wings, England Bingo players' arms or dinner ladies arms?

You need to stimulate the muscle tissue and hope your skin will follow. For post-menopausal women, you might experience your body shifting from having Gynoid fat displacement to Android fat displacement; you'll start seeing your arms gettin' smaller and your waist gettin' bigger! This is because of the loss of estrogen and other hormonal components that are changing in your body.

Due to the previous amounts of body fat stored in your arms, you now have extra skin hanging around because the fat is gone. The best thing to do is to 'say your prayers' and start doing some arm work. Swimming and Aqua-jogging are great too as they to have a circumferential impact on your arms.

Great Exercises for your Arms, See **Bi, Tri** in Exercise Reference Section

1. Biceps curl: Dumbells or bands 2-3 sets 12-20 reps moderate/light weight
2. Triceps Extension: Dumbells, 2-3 sets, 12-20 reps moderate/light weight
3. Assisted Pull Ups: with a Machine 2x's, 6-10 reps
4. Wide Grip Lat pull down 2x's, 6-10 Reps, Lighter Weight
5. Military Press: Dumbells or a Machine, 2-3 Sets, 8-10 reps, light/moderate weight (This will also help build spinal density which also reduces the risk of osteoporosis)

Question #4: Help! My boobs are saggy; is it possible to lift them without surgery?

Yes, it's definitely possible! You need to build up the muscle under the fat to help perk and lift. It needs to be all over, so doing a whole bunch of pushups isn't going to cut it.

Refer also to the Exercise Reference Section for more **Upper Body/Chest (Tri, Bi, C)** Exercises.

1. Incline chest press 2-3 sets, 6-15 reps, moderate-heavy weight
2. Decline chest press 2-3 sets, 6-15 reps, moderate weight
3. Flat bench Dumbell Flies 2-3 sets, 10-15 reps, moderate-light weight
4. Cable Crossovers 2 sets, 6-10 reps, moderate-light weight
5. Hand Compression Drill, hold for 20-30sec, repeat 2-3x's
6. Seated Fly, generally called a "peck deck" machine, 2-3 sets, 6-12 reps, moderate weight.

1. Are you ever too old to exercise?

No, exercise is VITAL to the elderly! It helps their bones stay dense, muscles stay strong, and it keeps their cardiovascular system working well. It also positively affects "Proprioception" skills, (neurological awareness to the surrounding environment).

A significant cause of death in the elderly is a suppressed immune system; brought on by a bone fracture (usually caused by a fall). When a bone breaks, the immune system has to work overtime to heal the damaged site, but it can only cope with so much. Pneumonia and other sicknesses can be deadly to a weakened immune system.

Proprioception skills help prevent those falls from ever happening!

Chapter 10

Exercise Equipment

If you have access to a good gym, it is more cost effective to use their facilities, as workout equipment is expensive, but for those of you who want to invest in exercise equipment, here are a few guidelines to get you on your way.

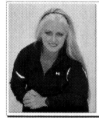 **Christin's Tip!**

You don't have to spend a fortune on fitness equipment to get in shape. Your best resources are at zero or minimal cost and can be found right outside your front door! So exercise outside and go swimming!

1. What do I really need and what do I want to spend?

What can you do outside instead of buying thousands of dollars worth of machinery? Here are some examples:

- **Treadmill**: If you do want to invest in a treadmill, it's better to go for one that best simulates running outside. When you run on the ground, you have to provide the forward force whereas on a treadmill, the belt is providing the forward motion, so you need to use the tilt facility to mimic the 'outside' effort. As you expect to run many miles (kilometers) on your treadmill, invest in quality otherwise you will end up with a bulking piece of unsightly furniture. Remember! Quality treadmills are very expensive whereas running outside is way better for you and is FREE!
- **Stationary/Spinning bike**: You have probably gathered by now that I prefer the great outdoors to working out inside. Doesn't matter to me if it's cold, raining or blowing a gale... outside beats inside any day! If you do like to go biking, how about getting yourself a nice road, bmx or mountain bike and go explore! Get the fresh air in your lungs and enjoy the benefits of training outside! If you still want a bike for working out indoors, go with quality...
- **Stair Stepper**: Hike, Bleachers, Roller blade, Snow board etc., there are many fun ways to completely tax your legs. Stair steppers are expensive and boring!

There are certain types of equipment that can't really be emulated outside and on those rainy lazy days, you might like to utilize.

A. **Elliptical/Cross trainer**: Make sure you get one that uses your arms and legs
B. **VersaClimber**: I have yet to use a harder piece of cardiovascular equipment that utilizes your entire body
C. **Dumbells and Barbells:** If you wanna lift old school style in the garage, more power to ya! Go for a barbell set and dumbbell rack as they're gonna be way cheaper and more functional than any bulking weight machine
D. **Heart Rate Monitor**: Without a doubt, this is the most important piece of equipment you could have, at least for the first 3 months

Here are some pieces of equipment that are inexpensive; you don't NEED them, but they have their uses!

Physioball: Low Cost, Is used to improve balance and stability

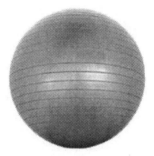

Bosu Ball: Medium Cost, used to improve balance and stability

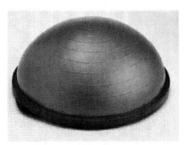

Bands: Very inexpensive, they can be used for multiple exercises. Very effective for females

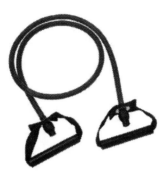

Medicine Balls: These are an awesome tool for assisting your plyometric work and getting your heart rate up. Very inexpensive and are GREAT for outdoor workouts!

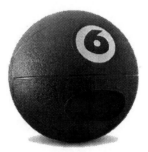

Jump Rope: Very inexpensive, Can be used to jack your heart rate up a different way for your superset or cardiovascular workout

I'm a great advocate for cardiovascular workouts in the fresh air. I have provided a choice of both indoor and outdoor workouts so you can exercise the way that suits you best.

Track Workouts

If you don't have access to a nearby track, get a pedometer to measure distance and find a surface that's comfortable to run on, e.g. gravel, grass, dirt.

- 400m is 1 lap around the track
- 200m is 1/2 lap around the track
- 100m is either a straight away segment or 1 curve segment
- 800m is 2 laps
- 1600m is 1 mile

Beginner

BASIC LEVEL I: Use a heart rate monitor if necessary. If you need to take a break or go slow, that's fine! If you can't finish the workout, it's ok! Work Up to it, then move on to the Basic II or Advanced Workout! Use the Exercise Reference Section (page 127) to demonstrate exercises.

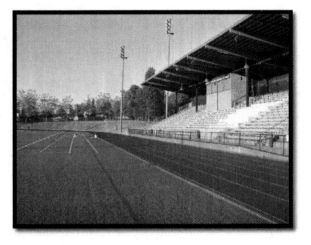

1. Walk 400m
2. Walk high knees 25m
3. Walk butt kicks 25
4. Side shuffle 15m quick down, 15m back (Face the same direction)
5. Speed Walk or jog 100m, walk back x5
6. Speed walk or jog 400m then RECOVER x 2-3
7. Use bleachers if the track has them, steps if not:

   - Walk up and down steps x5
   - Step Ups x8 each leg, 3 sets
   - Leg up/up down/downs
   - Side steps x12, 2 sets
   - Pushups x10, 2-3 sets
   - Triceps dips x10-15 2-3sets

- Full sit ups 30sx2

8. Walk or jog 400m
9. Stretch! 5-10min

Total: 1 1/2-1 3/4 Miles

BASIC LEVEL II

1. Jog 400m
2. Running high knees 25m
3. Running butt kicks 25
4. Side shuffle 15m quick down, 15m back (Face the same direction)
5. Faster Run 100m, walk back x5
6. Jog 400m then RECOVER
7. Run 200m x 3
8. Use bleachers if the track has them, steps if not:

   - Walk up and down steps x5
   - Step Ups x8 each leg 3 sets
   - Leg up/up down/downs
   - Side steps x12, 2 sets
   - pushups x10, 2-3 sets
   - triceps dips x10-15 2-3sets
   - full sit ups 30sx2

9. Walk or jog 400m
10. Stretch! 5-10min

Intermediate

1. Warm Up: Run 800m
2. High Knees 25m
3. Butt Kicks 25m
4. Side Shuffle 15m down and back, Face the same way
5. 800m Run x 2
6. 4x200m Sprint Timed, Try to keep the same pace
7. 2x400m Run with bleachers or stairs
8. 100m jog
9. Stretch! 5-10min

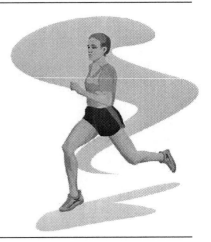

Total: 2 1/2 Miles

Advanced

This is a Mid-Distance Workout

1. Warm Up: Run 1600m
2. High Knees, Butt Kicks, Side Shuffle 1-2min
3. Run another 1600m
4. Run 400m fast x2
5. 4x200m Sprint Timed
6. 800m Run: Sprint Straight-aways, Jog Corners
7. Slow jog 200m
8. Walk 200-300m
9. Stretch

Total: A little over 3 1/2 miles

Pool Workouts

Pool workouts are effective for both swimmers and non-swimmers. If you can't swim right now, that's ok... get yourself an aqua belt. Follow the aqua jogging workouts, they'll help! Join a swim class or get a friend to teach you to swim, and before you know it you'll be swimming like the proverbial fish!

Aqua Jogging

Aqua jogging is a great way to get in the pool and have a great workout if you can't swim. Aqua jogging means running in the water. You use a floatable waist belt to keep you buoyant. Pools normally provide aqua belts and floaty weights, but if your local pool doesn't have one, any swim shop will... so get some! Aqua jogging is great because there's no pressure on your joints; it gets your heart rate up and really works your cardiovascular system! It's also great for rehabbing and injury and if you have any mobility ailments.

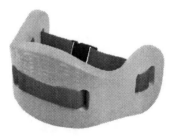

Aqua Belt

- *50m is 1 lap, down and back*
- *25m is just down, unless you are using a full sized Olympic pool; which is unlikely!*
- *You will be using the deep and shallow ends of the Pool!*

The Aqua Jog Workout

1. Aqua Jog 50m
2. Aqua Jog Knees Up 25m
3. Cross country Skier Back
4. Bicycle down 25m
5. Doggy Paddle Back
6. Aqua jog Down
7. Kick back
8. Tread water 30s, sprint down aqua belt 25m, when you get to the shallow end, jog, Recover then go back x3
9. Repeat 2x 1-9

Pool Workout with Weights

Lifting Weights in the pool is a great way to help strengthen your muscles without the impact that gravity brings! Think of it as a 360° workout because of the water pressure on your muscles; you'll feel it everywhere!

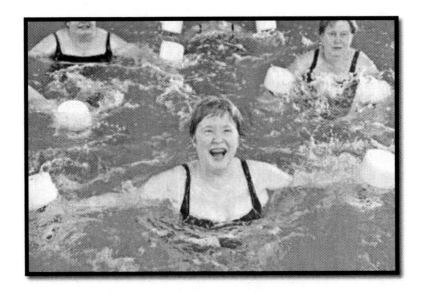

The Weights Workout!

1. Aqua Jog Knees Up 25m
2. Cross country Skier Back
3. Bicycle down 25m
4. Doggy Paddle Back
5. Aqua jog Down
6. Kick back
7. Tread water 30s, sprint down aqua belt 25m, when you get to the shallow end, jog, Recover then go back x3
8. Repeat 2x 1-8
9. Grab Floaty Weights: (6-10 reps each hand is fine, 2 sets)

   - Biceps Curl, Thumbs up
   - Back Row
   - Triceps extensions
   - Jumping Jacks
   - Fly
   - X-country Skier
   - Release the weights and kick 50m
   - Finish with Aqua Jogging 50m

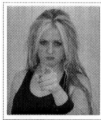 ## Christin's Rant!

When you workout, make sure you're actually working. I hate it when I see aerobic or pool classes that have a whole bunch of people just standing around...doing anything BUT working out! It doesn't help when the instructor is teaching horrible, non-moving exercises either. MOVE. MOVE YOUR BODY. KEEP MOVING. Slowly bouncing up and down and in the water does not a workout make!

If you want REAL changes, do REAL workouts!

Swimmers

Intermediate

- 50m is 1 lap, down and back
- 25m is just down, unless you are using a full sized Olympic pool; which is unlikely!

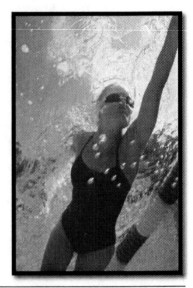

1. Swim 100m (2 laps)
2. Stretch
3. Your choice of Freestyle (crawl), backstroke or breaststroke, 250m x2
4. Swim Timed: 50mx3
5. Tread Water: 1min
6. Kick 50m
7. Finish 100m Easy

Advanced

1. Swim 100m (2 laps)
2. Stretch
3. 16 laps, 800m
4. Kick 50m
5. Swim timed sprints 50m x3
6. Tread Water 1min
7. Kick 50m
8. Finish 200m Easy

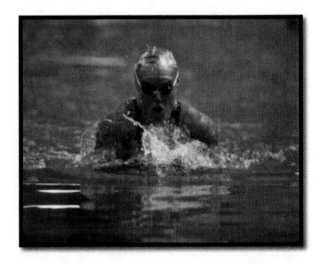

Exercise Reference

Back: B

Barbell Back Row – B1

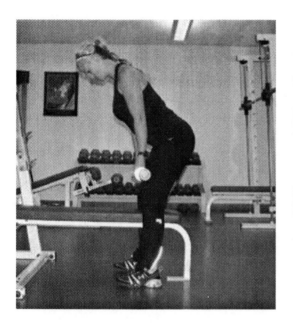 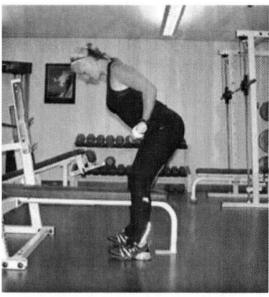

- Chest Out
- Stay Retracted
- Elbows in tight
- Hands Face Up
- Keep Core Tight
- Slight bend in hips and knees
- Drop Upper Body down

- Pull towards your Belly Button
- Keep a tight core and back
- Maintain spinal alignment
- Don't drop your chin down

Band Back Row – B2

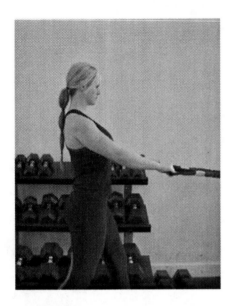 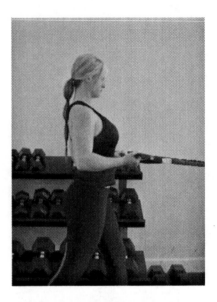

- Chest Out
- Extend shoulders out
- 1 Leg forward, 1 leg back
- Start with your hands facing down
- Keep Core Tight
- Retract...

- Then turn and pull
- Keep shoulders down, chest out
- You can do Single or Double Arms
- Squeeze below your shoulder blades, this is where you should feel it.

Bosu Band Back Row – B3

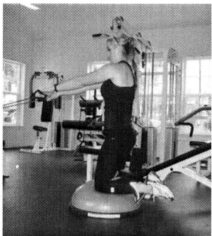

- Chest Out
- Extend shoulders out
- Both knees hip width apart on the Bosu
- Start with your hands facing down
- Keep Core Tight

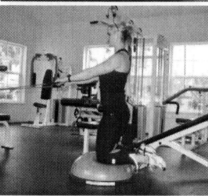

- Retract...
- Don't drop your head down

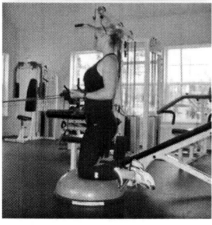

- Turn and pull
- Keep shoulders down, chest out
- You can Do Single Arms or Doubles
- Squeeze below your shoulder blades, this is where you should feel it.

Heavy Dumbell Back Row – B4

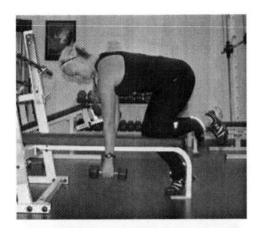

- Fully extend at the Shoulder joint
- Left knee up, rt leg down, or vice versa
- Keep opposite arm directly underneath shoulder joint
- Keep back flat

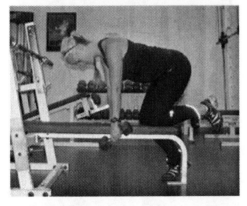

- Retract
- Chest goes out
- Shoulders go down

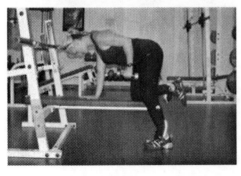

- Stay Retracted
- Pull arms down so the bar is slightly above your chest
- Exhale
- DO NOT pull the bar lower than your chest

Narrow Grip Lat Pull – B5

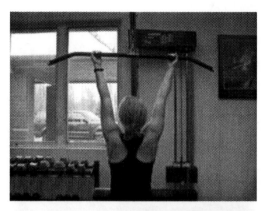

- Place hands shoulder width apart or slightly wider
- Fully extend at the shoulder joint
- Inhale

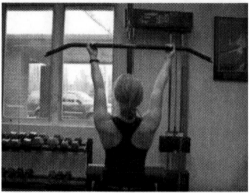

- Retract
- Chest goes out
- Shoulders go down

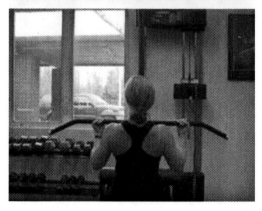

- Stay Retracted
- Pull arms down so the bar is slightly above your chest
- Exhale
- DO NOT pull the bar lower than your chest

Wide Grip Lat Pull Down – B6

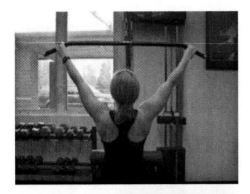

- Keep hands out wide
- Fully extend at the shoulder joint

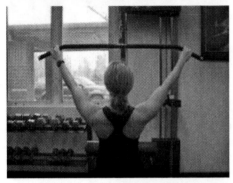

- Retract
- Keep your chest up

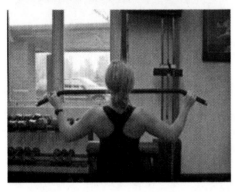

- Pull so the bar comes to your chin
- Use lighter weight

Retraction Exercises – B7

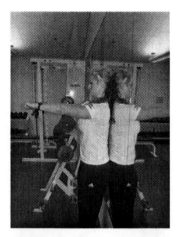 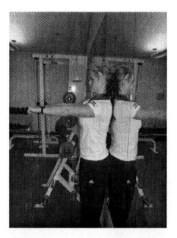

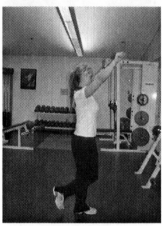 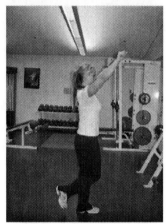

- EXTENDED PICTURES
- Go Up against a mirror and fully extend at the shoulder joint, forward
- Or, keep your arms fully extended upwards...

- RETRACTED PICTURES
- Then stick your chest out and flatten your shoulders up against the mirror
- Keep your shoulders down
- Then for the incline move, bring shoulders down

Walking Back Row – B8

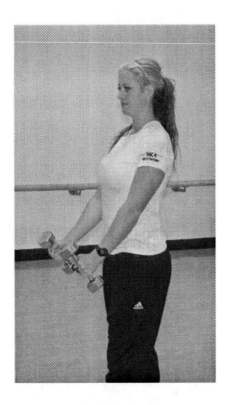

- Keep back straight
- Arms extended
- Elbows in tight

- Extend your arms back to 90°
- Single or double arms

Machine Back Row – B9

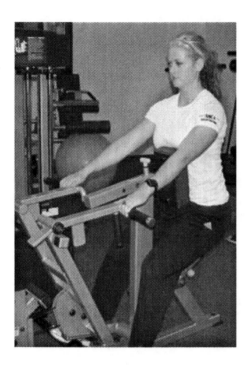 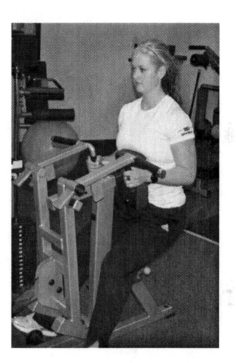

- Hands can face either down, up or neutral
- Chest up Shoulders back
- Eyes straight ahead

- Pull back
- Your arms should be parallel to your chest
- Keeping chest out
- Pause and hold
- Exhale as you return to the start position

Bosu Ball: BB

Bosu Bands Chest Press – BB1

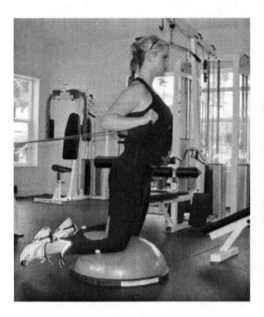 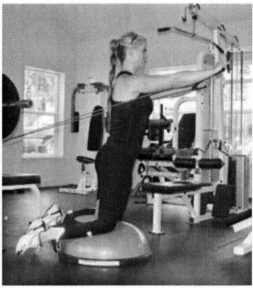

- Chest Out
- Shoulders Back
- Elbows at 45°
- Both knees on Bosu, hip width apart
- Use your chest not your shoulders
- Keep Core Tight! You can have the band at an angle as an Incline Chest Press, or you can have it level, as a Flat Chest Press

- Keep your Feet off the ground
- Fully extend your arms
- Slightly lean into the motion
- You can Do Single Arms or Doubles
- Still stay tight

Bosu Band Back Row – BB2

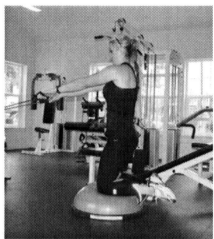

- Chest Out
- Extend shoulders out
- Both knees hip width apart on the bosu
- Start with your hands facing down
- Keep Core Tight

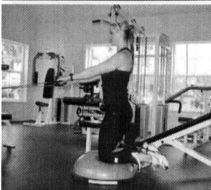

- Retract...
- Don't drop your head down

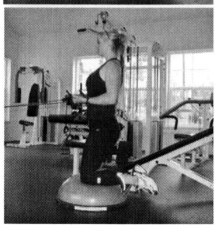

- Turn and pull
- Keep shoulders down, chest out
- You can Do Single Arms or Doubles
- Squeeze below your shoulder blades, this is where you should feel it.

Bosu Ab Hold – BB3

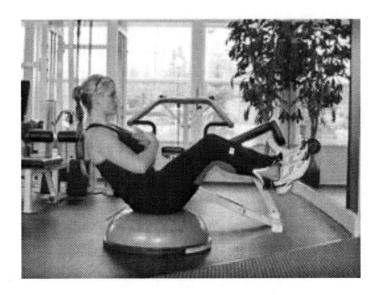

- Sit in the middle of the Bosu
- Lean back slightly
- Keep your knees up and hold

Bosu Full Sit Up – BB4

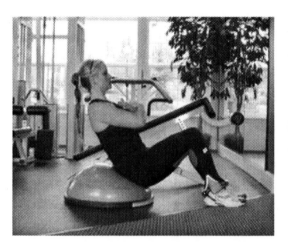 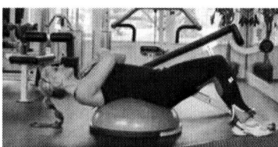

- Lie Down on the Bosu
- Have your hands across your chest
- Keep your feet on the ground

- Slowly Reach Back past 180°
- Exhale as you come up
- Don't sit up all the way, have tension on your Abs the whole time

Bosu Plank Hold – BB5

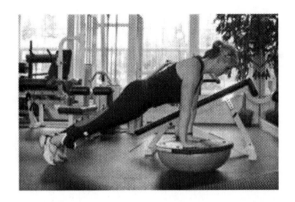 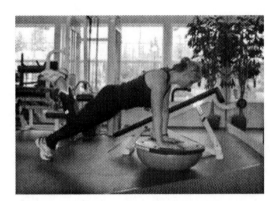

- Place your hands shoulder width apart on the Bosu, face them forward
- Get in a Plank Hold position
- Stay on the balls of your Feet
- Keep your butt down, don't sag your Lower Back

- You can make this exercise harder by lifting up 1 Leg, Moving your Arms side to side or forward and backwards

Bosu Squat – BB6

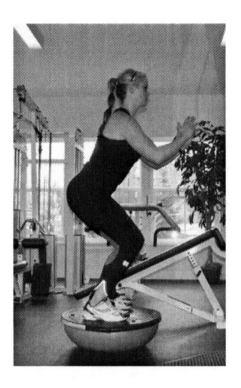 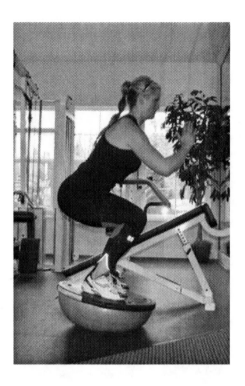

- Keep feet hip width apart
- Slight bend in knees
- Keep hips back
- Chest out, shoulders back, stay retracted
- Stay in the Middle of the Bosu
- You can put 1 foot on and then step onto the Bosu, or you can jump onto it

- As you keep your hips back, lower down to 90°
- Keep Back straight
- As you stand back up, focus on having stability-little movement
- You can make this harder by moving your legs side to side or forwards and backwards-staying down

Biceps: Bi

Band Biceps Curl – Bi1

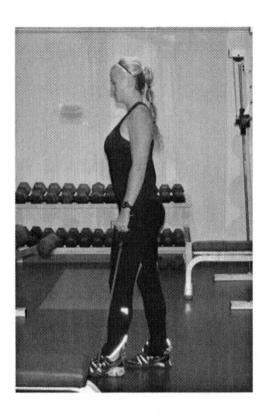 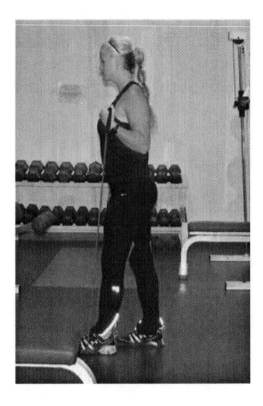

- Chest Out
- Shoulders Back
- Elbows In Tight
- Arms Down
- Keep Core Tight
- Stay Retracted

- Turn Hands
- Arms Come all the Way Up
- Stay Tight with your Retracted shoulders and Back
- Keep Elbows In
- You can Do Single Arms or Doubles

Curl Turn Press – Bi2

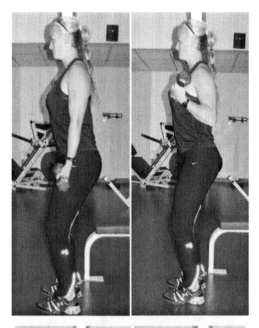

- Start Biceps Curl, arms full extended
- Shoulders out chest back (Retracted)
- Slight bend in the hips

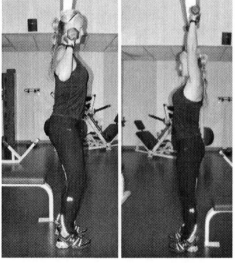

- Curl
- Elbows in tight
- Turn, turn hands around and lift to above shoulder joint
- Finish w/a straight press

Negative Biceps Curl – Bi3

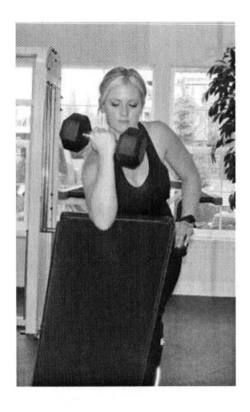 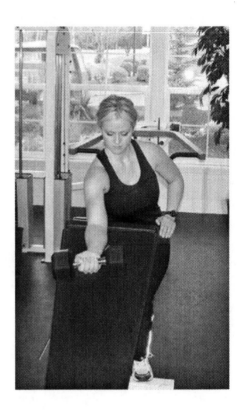

- Find a bench that has a sharp decline in it: i.e: preacher curl rack, decline bench, incline bench
- Keep your shoulder back
- Use heavy weight and go slow on the way down for
- about a 6-8 second count

- You can use your opposite hand to help your mover arm up Repeat 3-4 Times

Physioball Biceps Curl – Bi4

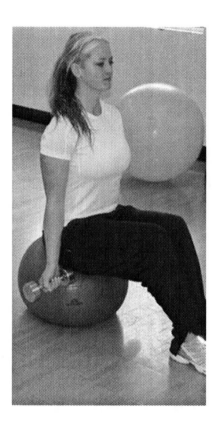 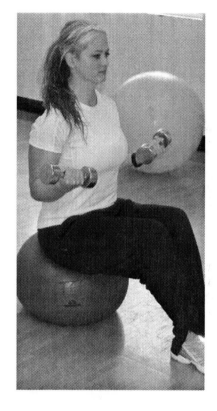

- Keep knees together
- Keep feet together
- Keep arms fully extended
- Chest out
- Shoulders back
- Stabilize the ball before any movement
- Inhale

- Curl and exhale
- Arms go straight up, keeping hands straight up
- Keeping knees and feet TOGETHER

Chest: C

45° Bench Press – C1

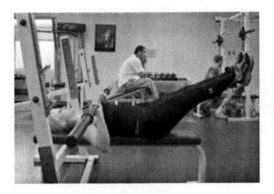 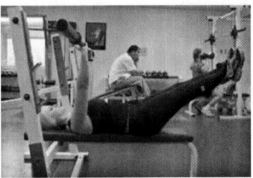

- Keep legs at 45 Degrees
- Keep legs straight
- Keep elbows at 45 Degrees
- Do NOT do if you have any back problems
- Do NOT do until at least 1 month into training

- Exhale as you press
- Lock your arms out
- Keep belly button down

Push Ups – C2

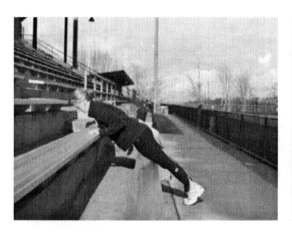 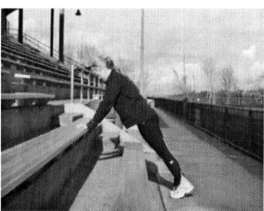

- Keep Body straight
- Hands slightly outside of shoulders
- Hands directly underneath your chest
- Elbows in tight
- Stay on your toes

- Exhale as you push up
- Maintain a straight body
- Keeping your butt down

Band Chest Press – C3

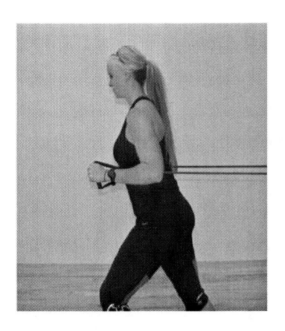 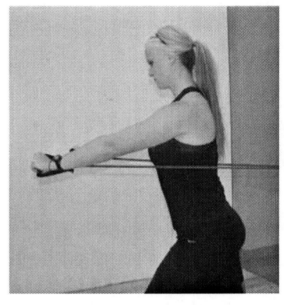

- Chest Out
- Shoulders Back and at 90°
- 1 Leg forward, 1 leg back
- Use your chest not your shoulders
- Arms Straight and in alignment with the band height
- Keep Core Tight
- Stay Retracted

- Fully extend your arms
- Slightly lean into the motion
- You can Do Single Arms or Doubles

Incline Dumbell Bench Press – C4

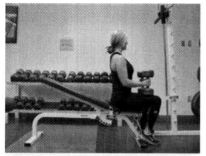

- Start off with the weights on your knees
- Bring your knee up with the weight

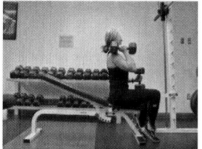

- Transfer the weight so your shoulders are supporting each dumbbell
- Inhale

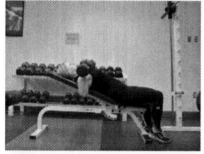

- Lie down
- Transfer dumbells into position-either facing forward, neutral or at 45°

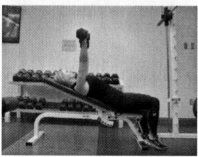

- Exhale as you press up
- Keeping the small of your back flat
- Lock your arms out
- Make sure you press from your chest, NOT your shoulders

Knee Push Ups – C5

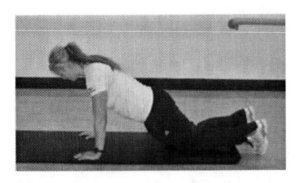

- Knees on floor
- Hands slightly outside of shoulders
- Hands directly underneath your chest

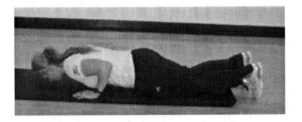

- Lower your body
- Keep belly button in
- Do not sag your lower back
- Nose comes close to touching ground

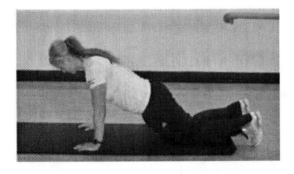

- Exhale as you push up
- Keeping your butt down

Machine Bench Press – C6

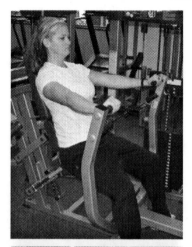

- Keep your arms out
- Shoulders down
- Chest out
- Hands where comfortable
- Inhale

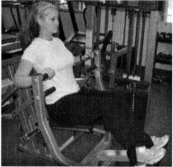

- Maintain a tight back
- Slowly allow bars to travel back
- DO NOT shrug your shoulders
- Go down far enough so your hands are even with your chest, but do not go back ANY farther-this can hurt your shoulders

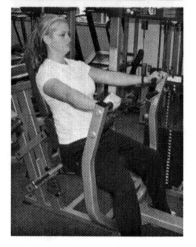

- Exhale as you press forward to the start position

Physioball Dumbell Chest Fly – C7

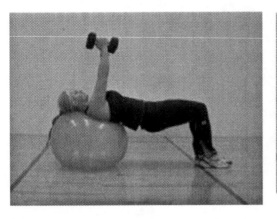 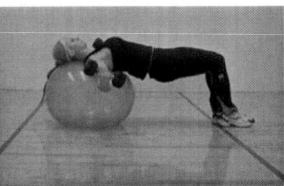

- Keep your feet and knees together
- Lift your butt up high and keep it tight
- Place your hands so they are facing each other
- Keep your head on the ball

- Reach out to the sides with your Arms
- Keep a slight bend in your Arms
- Pretend like you are give a bear hug to someone
- Keep your shoulders down as your bring your hands back together

Physioball Dumbell Chest Press – C8

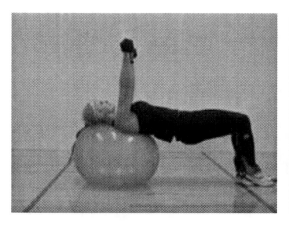 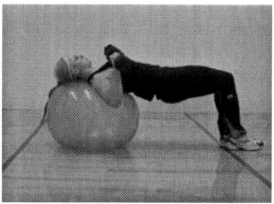

- Keep your feet and knees together
- Lift your butt up high and keep it tight
- Place your hands so the thumbs face each other
- Keep your head on the ball

- Lower arms down so your elbows are at 90°
- Keep arms at 45°
- Keep shoulders down
- Squeeze your abs and exhale as you Press back up

Physioball Dumbell Plank Hold/and or Roll – C9

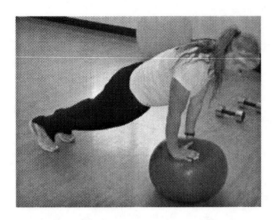

- Keep hands directly underneath your chest on the ball
- Keep your back straight
- Keep your butt down

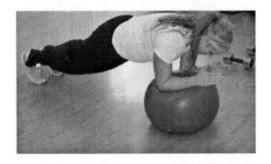

- Gently roll down onto your elbows maintaining a tight back and waist
- Keep hands straight forward

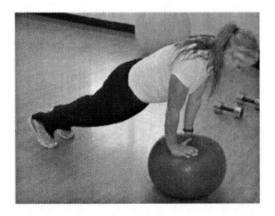

- Exhale as you use your arm and shoulder strength to move yourself back up to the start position
- Keep your butt down

Push Up Pop Offs – C10

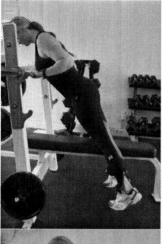

- Keep feet hip width apart
- Keep legs straight
- Lower your upper body to where the bar is below your chest
- Chest out, shoulders back, stay retracted
- Keep Elbows in TIGHT! They should be touching your Lats-(sides)

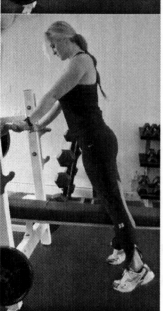
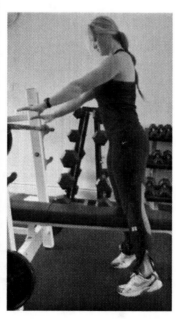

- Drive off as you fully extend your arms
- Keep body straight, butt in tight
- Don't sag your lower back

Up Up Down Downs - C11

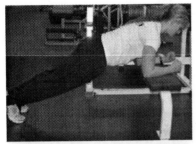

- Keep back straight
- Arms both at 90°
- Elbows in tight

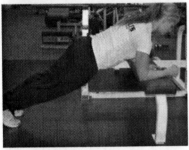

- Come up on one hand...

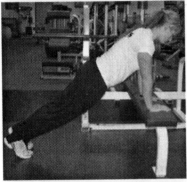

- Then the other...

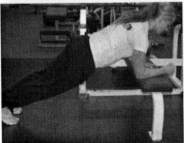

- Come down on the same arm you started with
- Keep your butt down

Barbell Bench Press – C12

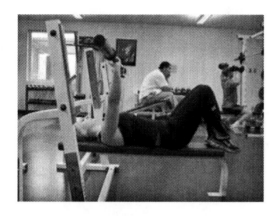 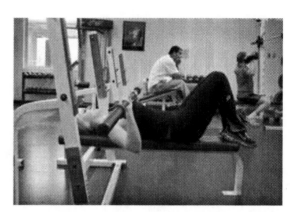

- Lay on your back
- Hold the bar so when you go down, your elbows should be at 90°
- I like to keep my feet UP on the bench
- Keep the small of your back down
- Keep your thumbs AROUND the bar
- Inhale

- Allow the bar to travel down to your chest
- Control the movement
- Your elbows should finish at 45°
- Exhale as you press back up to the start position

Bosu Bands Chest Press – C13

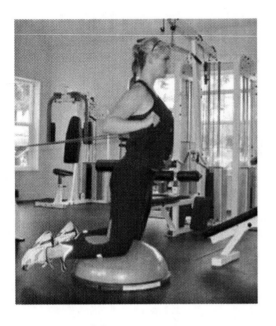 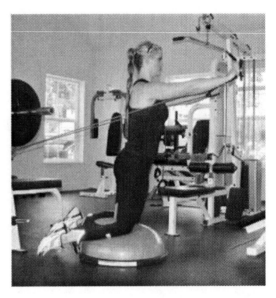

- Chest Out
- Shoulders Back
- Elbows at 45°
- Both knees on Bosu, hip width apart
- Use your chest not your shoulders
- Keep Core Tight! You can have the band at an angle as an Incline Chest Press, or you can have it level, as a Flat Chest Press

- Keep your Feet off the ground
- Fully extend your arms
- Slightly lean into the motion
- You can Do Single Arms or Doubles
- Still stay tight

Core, CR

Basic Crunch - CR1

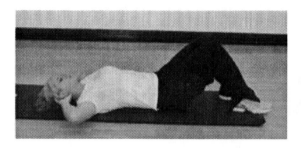 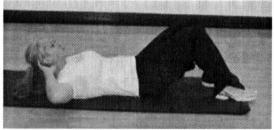

- Lay on your Back
- Legs Bent
- Feet Flat
- Inhale

- Belly Button goes down towards the ground
- Hips come up
- Gently lift your head up toward the ceiling
- Hold
- Then Release
- Exhale

Bosu Ab Hold – CR2

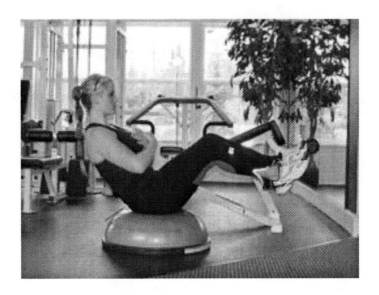

- Sit in the middle of the Bosu
- Lean back slightly
- Keep your knees up and hold

Bosu Full Sit Up – CR3

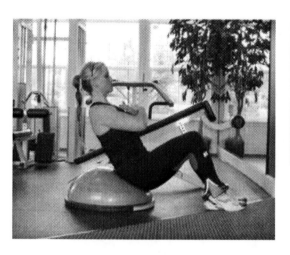
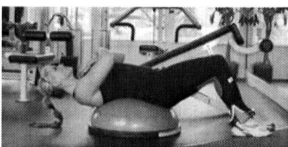

- Lie Down on the Bosu
- Have your hands across your chest
- Keep your feet on the ground

- Slowly Reach Back past 180°
- Exhale as you come up
- Don't sit up all the way, have tension on your Abs the whole time

Bosu Plank Hold – CR4

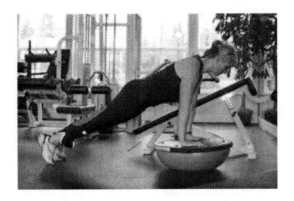 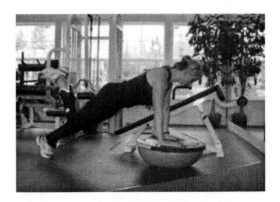

- Place your hands shoulder width apart on the Bosu, face them forward
- Get in a Plank Hold position
- Stay on the balls of your Feet
- Keep your butt down, don't sag your Lower Back

- You can make this exercise harder by lifting up 1 Leg, Moving your Arms side to side or forward and backwards

Full Sit Up – CR5

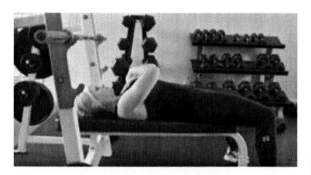 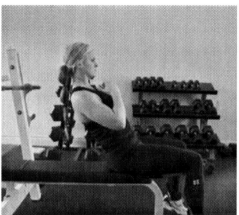

- Lie Down on the Floor or a Bench
- Have your hands across your chest

- Exhale as you come up to a little less than 90°
- Do NOT hold on to anything with your feet

Physioball Crunch – CR6

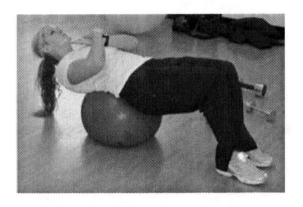 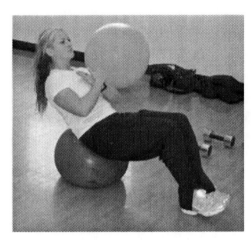

- Keep knees together
- Keep feet together
- Keep Back slightly bent back-Abdominal wall fully extended
- Stabilize the ball before any movement
- Inhale
- Hands cross the chest or supporting the neck

- Keep back straight as you lift
- Stop right before you have no more tension

Physioball Plank Hold/and or Roll - CR7

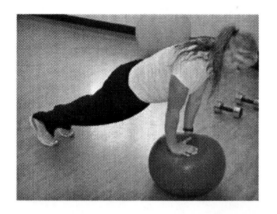

- Keep hands directly underneath your chest on the ball
- Keep your back straight
- Keep your butt down

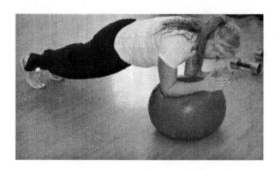

- Gently roll down onto your elbows maintaining a tight back and waist
- Keep hands straight forward

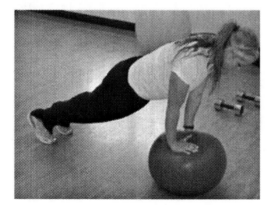

- Exhale as you use your arm and shoulder strength to move yourself back up to the start position
- Keep your butt down

Plank Hold on Hands – CR8

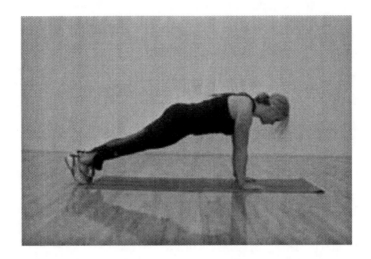

- Keep your Body and Back Straight
- Put your Hands facing Forward
- Keep Neck and Head in Spinal Alignment
- Stay on Toes
- Do not sag your Lower Back

Side Crunch – CR9

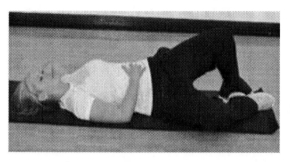 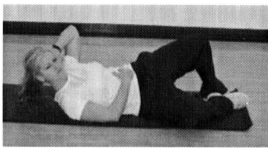

- Keep hips slightly rotated away from the direction that you are working
- Place the hand of the side you are working behind your head, the opposite on your stomach
- Keep the knee of the side you are working up and the opposite down towards the mat

- Crunch and turn slightly up
- Bring hips back a bit toward your elbow
- exhale

Up Up Down Downs - CR10

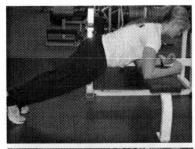

- Keep back straight
- Arms both at 90°
- Elbows in tight

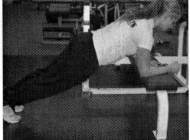

- Come up on one hand...

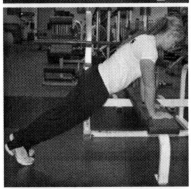

- Then the other...

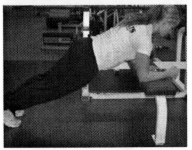

- Come down on the same arm you started with
- Keep your butt down

Barbell Crunch Butt Lift – CR11

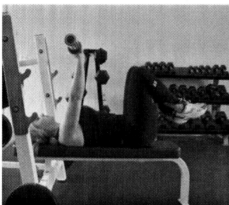

- Lie on Back
- Pick up Barbell and position it as you would a chest press
- Legs up

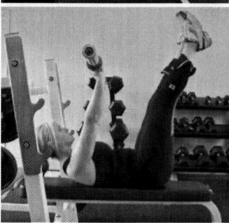

- Crunch Up, extend your legs
- Keep Belly Button down
- You can add a chest press if you so desire
- Lift Your Hips up off the bench for a butt life
- Do not do this if you have a weak back
- Keep head back
- Arms still fully extended

Full Sit up to Jump – CR12

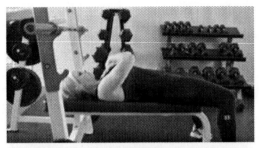

- Lie Down on the Floor or a Bench
- Have your hands across your chest

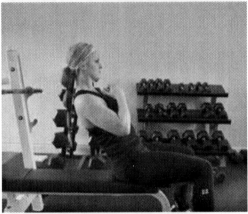

- Exhale as you come up to a little less than 90°
- Do NOT hold on to anything with your feet

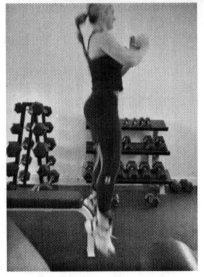

- Keeping your feet hip width apart, Jump up into the air
- Use your arms: drive them back then up into the air
- Land, and lie back down, Repeat

(JHR) Jack Your Heart Rate: J

High Knee Skips – J1

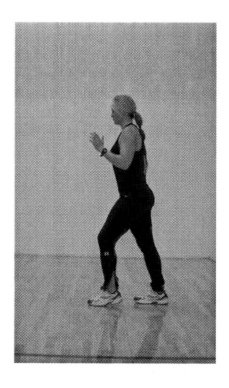
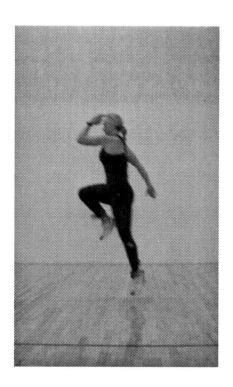

- 1 Leg forward, 1 Leg Back
- Lean Forward slightly

- Drive your knee up in the air as you skip
- Opposite Arm Goes up
- Opposite Leg
- Try to get off the ground as high as possible

High Knees –J2

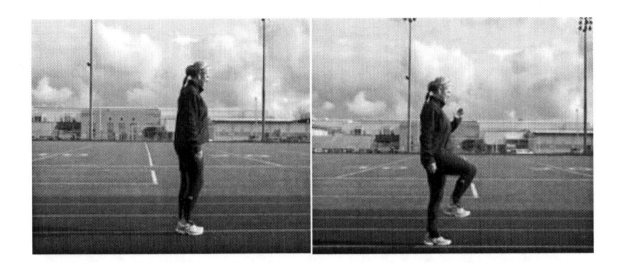

- Keep back straight

- Bring knee up high to 90° angle
- Keep foot flexed (keep toe up)
- Move arms up opposite to your legs
- Then switch
- Is performed walking or running

Butt Kicks – J3

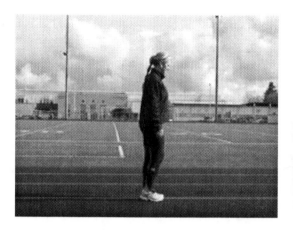 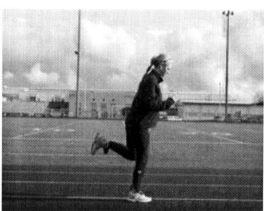

- Keep back straight

- Kick 1 leg up towards butt
- The purpose of this exercise is to warm up the hamstring (the back of the leg)
- Opposite arm move with kicking leg, to 45-90°
- These can be done walking or running

Mountain Climbers – J4

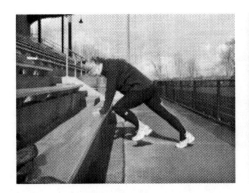 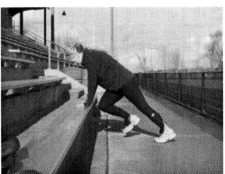

- Keep back straight
- Stand on 1 leg

- Kick 1 leg up towards butt
- The purpose of this exercise is to warm up the hamstring (the back of the leg)
- Opposite arm move with kicking leg, to 45-90°
- These can be done walking or running

Legs: L

Abductor Machine – L1

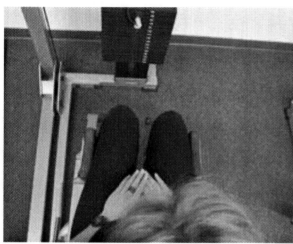 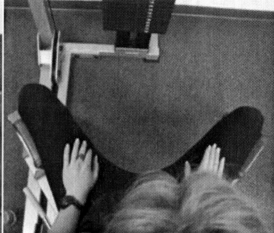

- Legs Start all the way in
- Chest out shoulders back
- Inhale

- Legs go all the way out
- Exhale

Adductor Machine – L2

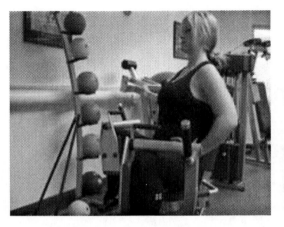 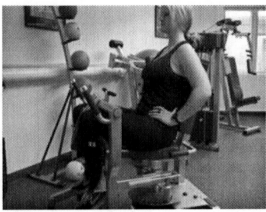

- Start with legs OUT
- Inhale
- Chest out Shoulders back

- Bring Legs in
- Exhale

At the Track High Knees – L3

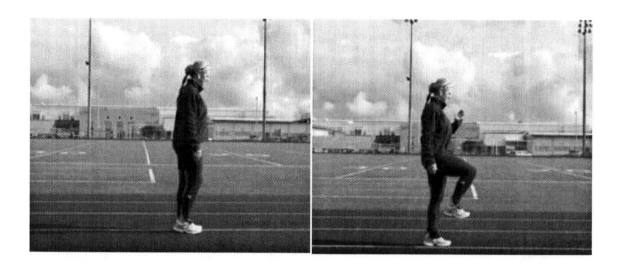

- Keep back straight

- Bring knee up high to 90° angle
- Keep foot flexed (keep toe up)
- Move arms up opposite to your legs
- Then switch
- Is performed walking or running

Butt Kicks – L4

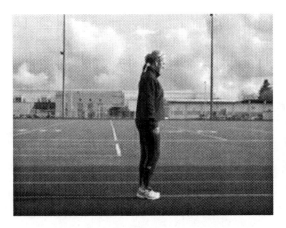 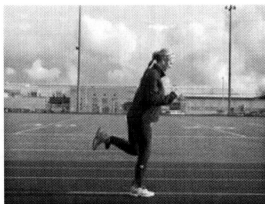

- Keep back straight

- Kick 1 leg up towards butt
- The purpose of this exercise is to warm up the hamstring (the back of the leg)
- Opposite arm move with kicking leg, to 45-90°
- These can be done walking or running

Barbell Squats – L5

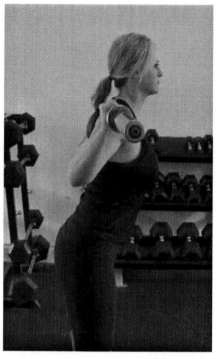 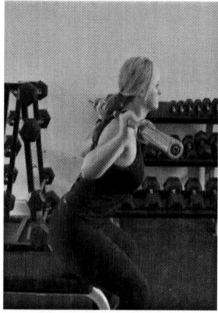

- Place the Bar below Axis Vertebrae
- Keep legs in a Plie position
- Chest and Eyes Stay Up
- Slight bend in hips

- Squat Down towards bench, keeping your back straight
- Keep Hips back
- Make sure your knees do not come forward
- Exhale as you stand back up
- You can sit down on the bench if you have difficulty keeping your hips back
- The pressure should be on your butt and thighs

Hamstring Curl – L6

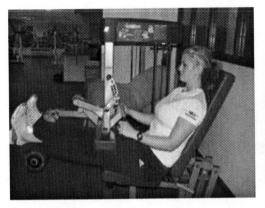 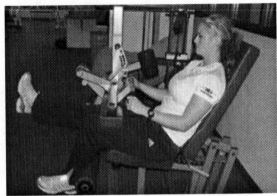

- Keep back straight
- Both Legs Up
- I like to use also the lying down hamstring curl machine
- Pad should rest directly below calf muscles
- Upper pad should be directly back behind and over your knee
- Your knee should be at the knobby axis of where the machine bends

- Curl down to a 90° angle hold, then back up

Long Lunge – L7

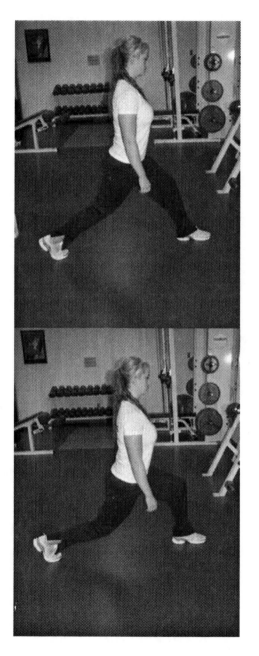

- Keep feet straight
- Take a big step so you engage the back of your front leg

- Lower hips straight down
- Do not allow your knee to come forward on your lead leg
- Do not allow your back knee to touch down
- Keep upper body slightly forward
- Exhale as you come back up
- Focus on contracting and working your lead leg glute, so in this photo, it would be my left glute and hamstring

Narrow Dumbell Squats – L8

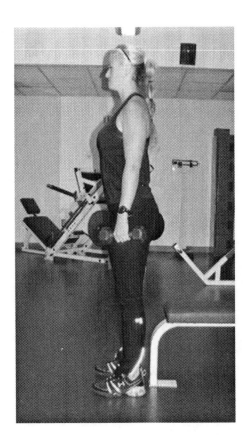 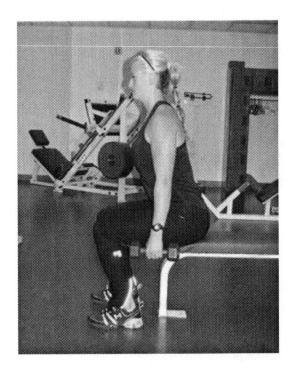

- Keep feet hip width apart
- Slight bend in knees
- Keep hips back
- Chest out, shoulders back, stay retracted

- As you keep your hips back, lower down to 90°
- Keep Back straight
- As you stand back up, focus on using the front part of your thighs, the Quadriceps

Narrow Leg Press – L9

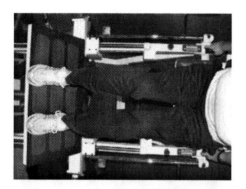

- Keep feet hip width apart
- Keep feet straight
- Keep knees in the same direction as feet

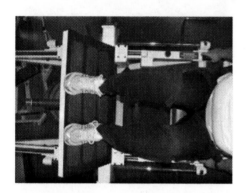

- Lower legs
- Focus on using your glutes and hamstrings-(your butt and back of legs)

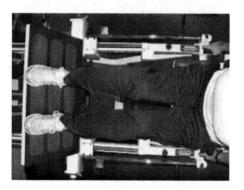

- Exhale as you push back
- Keep your butt down

Pickers Basic – L10

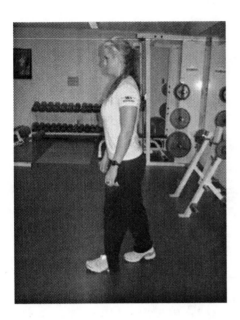 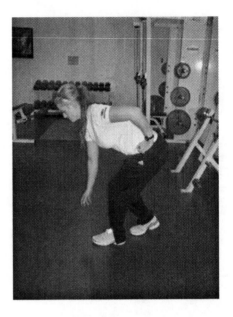

- Keep 1 leg forward 1 leg back
- Keep both feet straight
- Keep hips back
- Back leg is used for support in balancing
- Do not put weight on the back leg

- Bend at the hip joint not back
- Keep your hips back
- Keep your back straight
- You should feel a slight pull on whatever leg is in front and you should feel the pull on the back of the leg and glute
- Pretend like you are "picking" something up off the ground

Pickers Advanced – L11

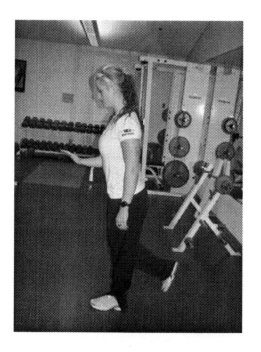
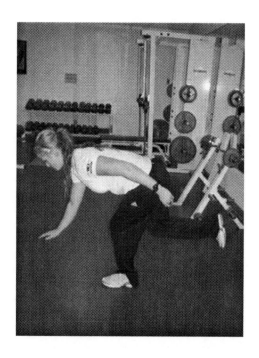

- Keep both feet straight
- Find your balance

- Bend at the hip joint
- Keep back straight
- Keep slight bend in your knee
- Pretend you are reaching forward to pick something up off the ground
- Center of gravity should be over your lead leg

Plie Hops – L12

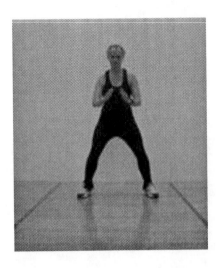
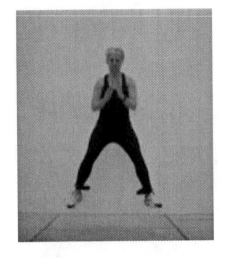

- Legs out wide
- Keep feet in the direction of your knees
- Keep hips back
- Arms start together, and then swing them back...

- Drive your arms Up in the air
- Jump off the ground
- Use your inner and outer thighs to generate power
- Land in the start position

Plie Squat or Wide Squat – L13

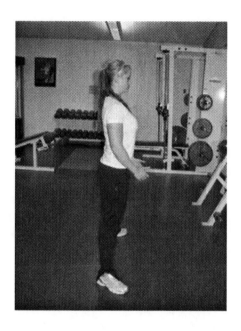 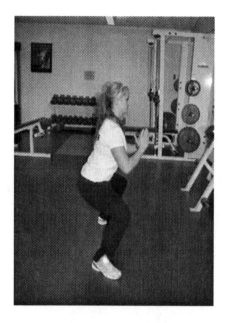

- Keep legs out past hips
- Keep feet in the same direction as knees

- Sit your butt BACK NOT forward
- Use a chair if necessary
- Keep knees in alignment with feet
- Keep your back straight
- Make sure you have covered your bases by doing a muscular imbalance assessment first. You should not be doing this exercise if your knees move or if your back sways out or has problems

Quadriceps Extension – L14

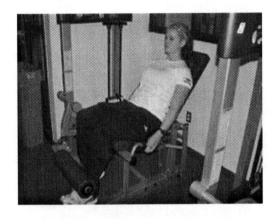 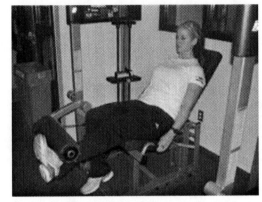

- Keep back straight
- Both Legs Down
- Pad should rest directly below calf muscles
- Your knee should be at the knobby axis of where the machine bends

- Extend at the knee joint
- Do not FULLY extend, rather, have a slight bend in your leg
- Hold slightly then lower

Single Leg Press – L15

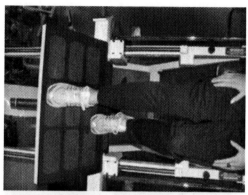

- Keep both feet straight
- Keep the foot of the leg that you are working up high as to impact the back of your legs
- Put the opposite leg down to support it, yet add no extra weight if possible
- You should not be doing this exercise if you have a muscular imbalance

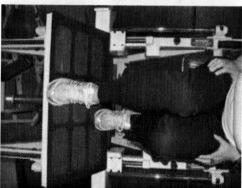

- Come forward to the machine
- Use your glutes and hamstrings
- You should be able to see the top ½ of your lead foot
- This exercise is used for stability and creating an equal balance of strength in each leg

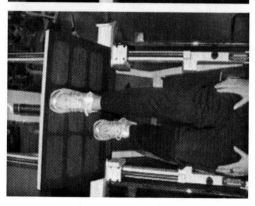

- Activate and press back with lead leg
- Exhale as your press back

Stationary Lunge Hop – L16

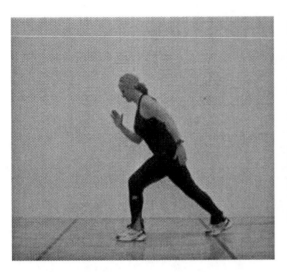 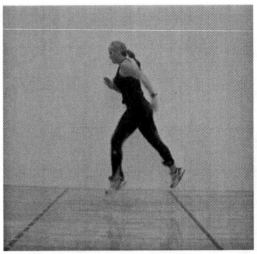

- Take a big long step, lead leg forward
- Lean forward slightly
- Opposite Hand goes forwards

- Drive up and Jump up in the air, bring up your lead knee
- Move both arms to help activate more potential power

Step Up – L17

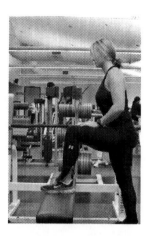

- Keep feet straight
- Keep lead foot all the way up on the bench
- Step up from your heel
- Keep hips back
- If you are just beginning, you can use a bench with less of an incline

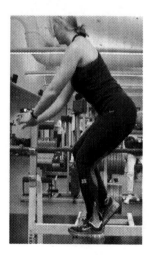

- Keep hips back
- Do not apply pressure to the helper leg
- You can step up and leave the lead leg up, or you can step down and take the lead leg off and repeat the process
- Focus on something in the ground to help you with

Wide Leg Press – L18

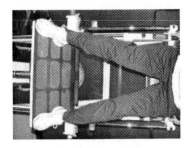

- Keep Feet in a Plie or Wide Squat position
- Keep knees in the same direction as feet

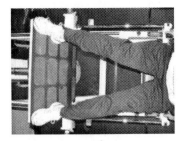

- Lower legs
- Focus on using your glutes and hamstrings-(your butt and back of legs)

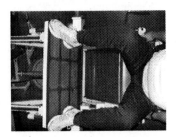

- Exhale as you push back
- Keep your butt down

Double Leg Jump – L19

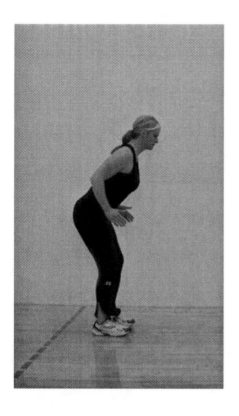 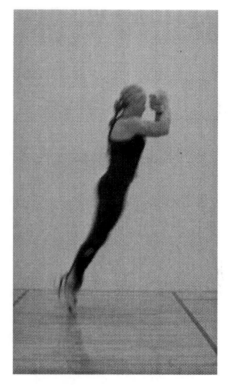

- Feet together, hip width apart
- Keep feet straight
- Lean Forward slightly
- Arms cock back to 90°
- Have your power come from your hips so keep your hips back

- Drive your arms Up in the air
- Fully extend your Body (this is called Triple Extension)
- Try to then bring your knees up after you jump
- Land in the start position

Calve Raise – L20

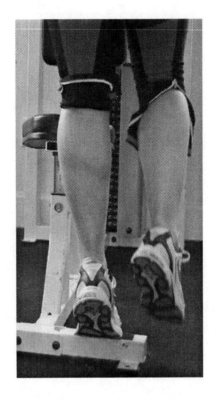

- Find a 90° Surface
- Go all the way down and up

Med Ball: M

Medball Chest Pass – M1

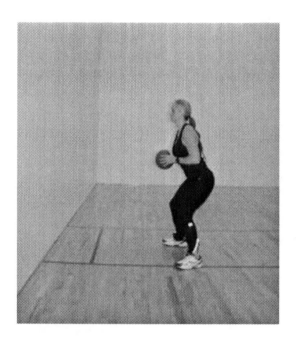
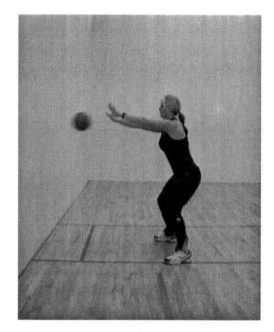

- Squat Down
- Keep Hips back
- Keep arms up
- The power comes from your hips not your arms, so use your hips!

- Fully extend your Arms
- Jump up off the ground if you desire
- Focus on using your chest and lower body to generate power
- Hips come slightly up as your Pass

Medball Toss Up – M2

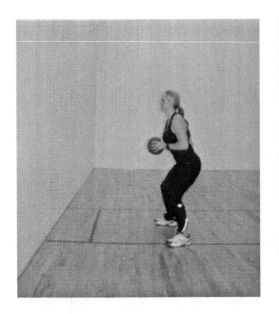 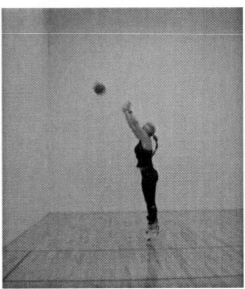

- Squat Down
- Keep Hips back
- Keep arms up
- The power comes from your hips not your arms, so use your hips!

- Extend your body up
- Jump up off the ground
- Throw the ball behind up and extend your arms forward
- Do not do if you have spine or back problems
- Be aggressive and drive/explode up as you throw

Medball Triceps Extension – M3

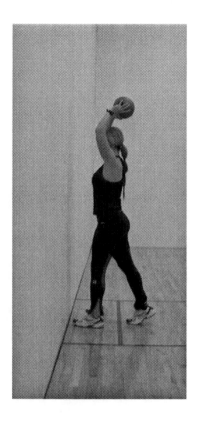 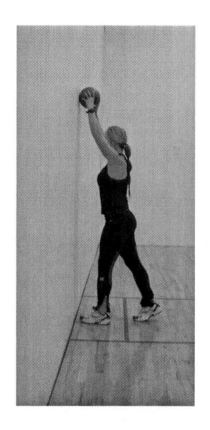

- 1 Leg forward, 1 Leg Back
- Extend your arms Up, holding onto the bal
- Use your Triceps and Core to throw the ball repeatedly against the wall
- Stare straight ahead

- Release the ball fast, catch and repeat

Behind the Head Throw – M4

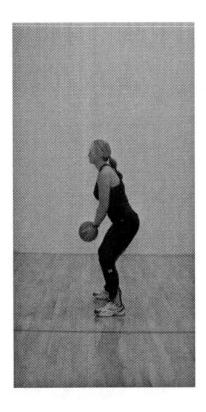 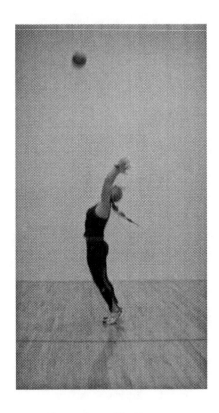

- Squat Down
- Keep Hips back
- Fully extend at the arm

- Extend your body up
- Jump up off the ground
- Throw the ball behind up and over your head
- Do not do if you have spine or back problems
- Be aggressive and drive/explode up as you throw

Physioball: PB

Physioball Dumbell Pullover – PB1

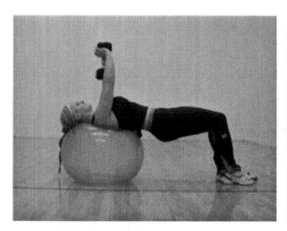 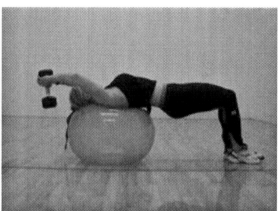

- Keep your feet and knees together
- Lie on the ball, so your Head is fully on the ball
- Make a triangle with your hands
- Hold the dumbell over your Chest

- Reach back with your arms
- Keep a slight bend in arms
- Pull back to start position using Lats

Physioball Biceps Curl – PB2

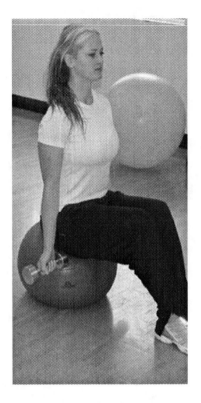 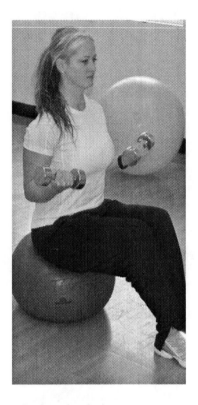

- Keep knees together
- Keep feet together
- Keep arms fully extended
- Chest out
- Shoulders back
- Stabilize the ball before any movement
- Inhale

- Curl and exhale
- Arms go straight up, keeping hands straight up
- Keeping knees and feet TOGETHER

Physioball Crunch – PB3

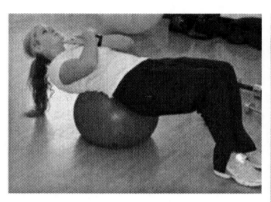 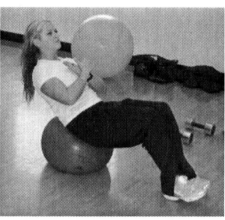

- Keep knees together
- Keep feet together
- Keep Back slightly bent back- Abdominal wall fully extended
- Stabilize the ball before any movement
- Inhale
- Hands cross the chest or supporting the neck

- Keep back straight as you lift
- Stop right before you have no more tension

Physioball Dumbell Chest Fly – PB4

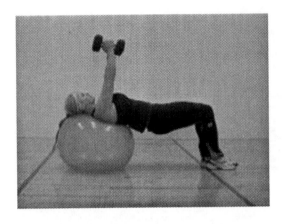 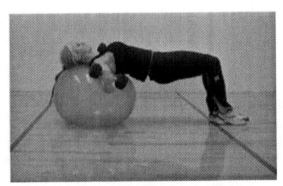

- Keep your feet and knees together
- Lift your butt up high and keep it tight
- Place your hands so they are facing each other
- Keep your head on the ball

- Reach out to the sides with your Arms
- Keep a slight bend in your Arms
- Pretend like you are give a bear hug to someone
- Keep your shoulders down as your bring your hands back together

Physioball Dumbell Chest Press – PB5

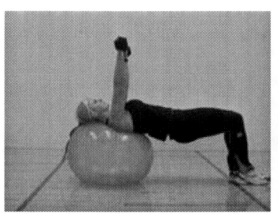 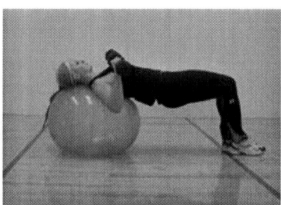

- Keep your feet and knees together
- Lift your butt up high and keep it tight
- Place your hands so the thumbs face each other
- Keep your head on the ball

- Lower arms down so your elbows are at 90°
- Keep arms at 45°
- Keep shoulders down
- Squeeze your abs and exhale as you Press back up

Physioball Plank Hold/and or Roll – PB6

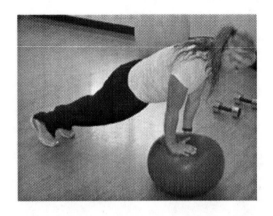

- Keep hands directly underneath your chest on the ball
- Keep your back straight
- Keep your butt down

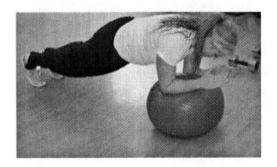

- Gently roll down onto your elbows maintaining a tight back and waist
- Keep hands straight forward

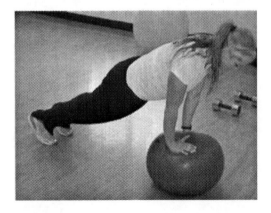

- Exhale as you use your arm and shoulder strength to move yourself back up to the start position
- Keep your butt down

Physioball Dumbell Shoulder Raise – PB7

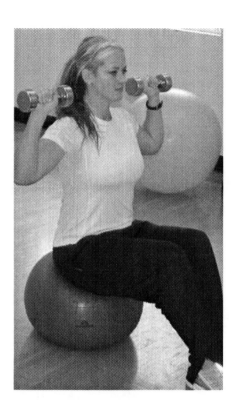 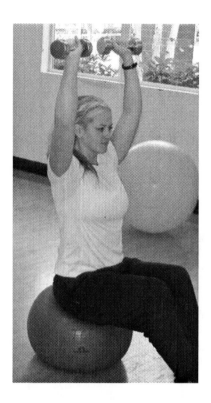

- Keep knees together
- Keep feet together
- Keep hands at 90°
- Chest out
- Shoulders back
- Stabilize the ball before any movement

- Press and exhale
- Fully extend at your arms
- Keeping knees and feet TOGETHER
- Go straight up not forward

Shoulders: S

Shoulder Raises – S1

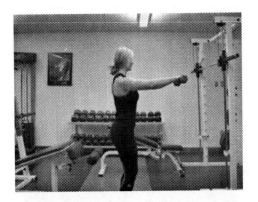

- Retract
- Chest out shoulders down
- Slight bend in the hips
- Arms slightly bent
- Single or double arm lift
- Then lower

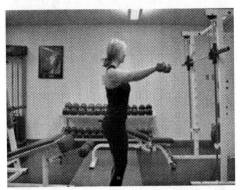

- Stay Retracted
- Chest out shoulders down
- Slight bend in the hips
- Arms slightly bent
- Single or double arm lift to 45° then lower

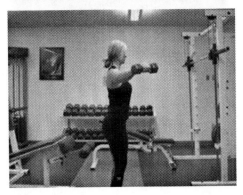

- Stay Retracted
- Chest out shoulders down
- Slight bend in the hips
- Arms slightly bent
- Single or double arm lift to 85-90° then lower

Heavy Shrugs – S2

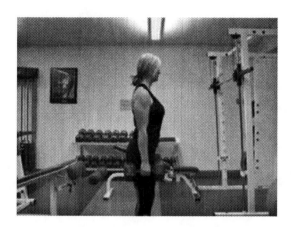 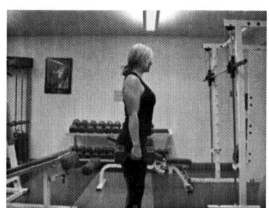

- Retract
- Slight bend in hips
- Feet slightly apart or hip width
- Relax your neck

- Stay Retracted
- Shrug shoulders straight up toward ceiling
- Do not roll shoulders
- Pause when you reach the top
- Exhale then lower

Machine Shoulder Raise – S3

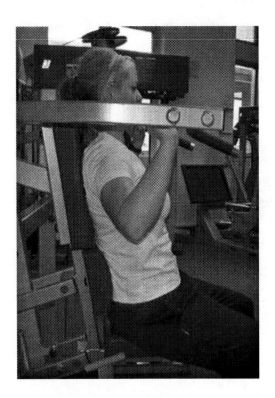 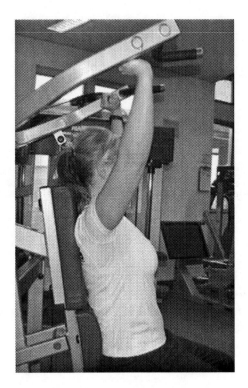

- Hands can face forward or neutral
- Chest up Shoulders back
- Eyes straight ahead
- Keep hands above your chest, NEVER at or lower as this would hurt your shoulders

- Press and exhale
- Fully extend at your arms
- Keeping Chest out

Physioball Dumbell Shoulder Raise – S4

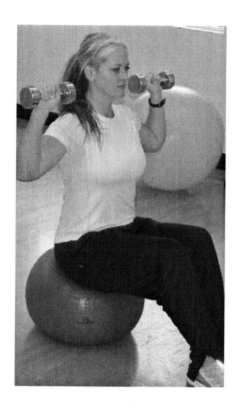 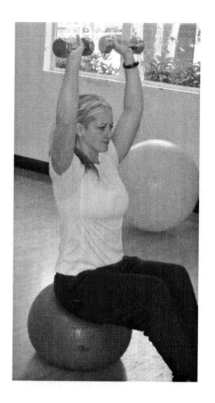

- Keep knees together
- Keep feet together
- Keep hands at 90°
- Chest out
- Shoulders back
- Stabilize the ball before any movement

- Press and exhale
- Fully extend at your arms
- Keeping knees and feet TOGETHER
- Go straight up not forward

Posterior Deltoid – S5

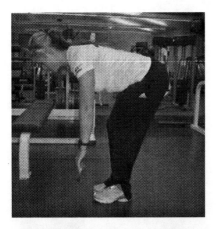

- Retract
- Hands face feet or each other
- Back straight and flat-spinal alignment
- Feet straight and close together

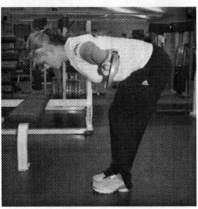

- Stay Retracted
- Lift arms up to 90° and pause hold
- Exhale as you lower arms to the start position
- Thumbs facing down

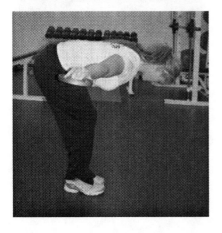

- Thumbs facing ahead

Walking Punch – S6

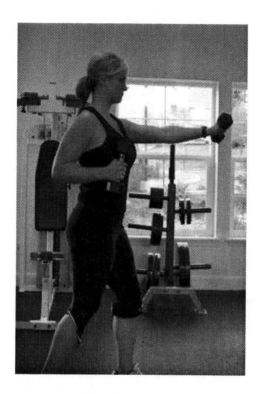

- As you walk, fully extend your arm out as a punch
- Keep your arm straight
- Keep the opposite arm at 90°
- Keep punching hand flat or thumbs up
- Keep Core tight

Walking Upper Cut – S7

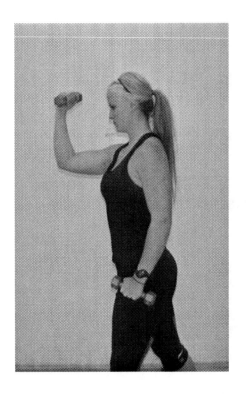 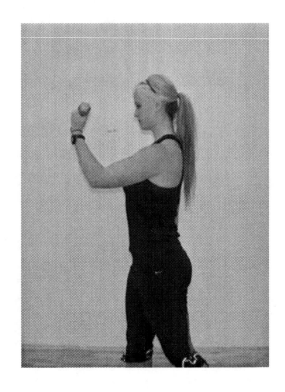

- While you walk, extend your hand up to create at least a 90° angle with your arm
- Keep your chest out
- Don't drop your other arm down, rather keep it at 90°

- Left leg forward, right arm up
- Right leg forward, left arm up

Upright Rows – S8

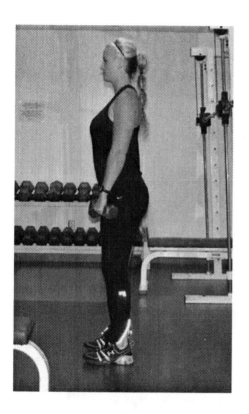 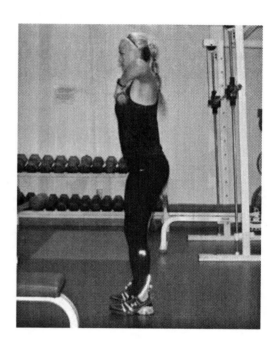

- Keep feet hip width apart
- Slight bend in knees
- Keep hips back
- Chest out, shoulders back, stay retracted
- Extend relaxed arms

- Lift your elbows up so they are higher than your hands
- Keep Back straight, Chest out
- Exhale as you come up

Track: T

High Knees – T1

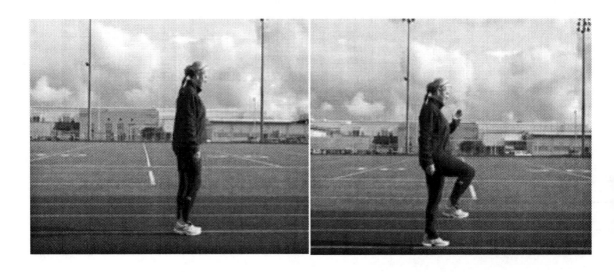

- Keep back straight

- Bring knee up high to 90° angle
- Keep foot flexed (keep toe up)
- Move arms up opposite to your legs
- Then switch
- Is performed walking or running

Butt Kicks – T2

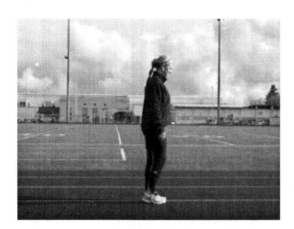 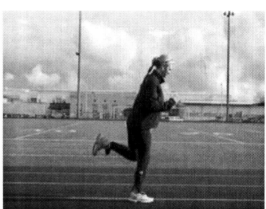

- Keep back straight

- Kick 1 leg up towards butt
- The purpose of this exercise is to warm up the hamstring (the back of the leg)
- Opposite arm move with kicking leg, to 45-90°
- These can be done walking or running

Mountain Climbers – T3

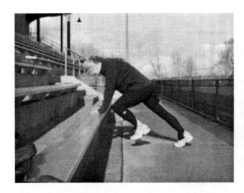 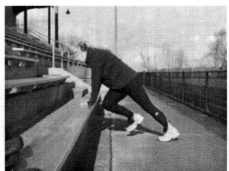

- Keep back straight
- Stand on 1 leg

- Kick 1 leg up towards butt
- The purpose of this exercise is to warm up the hamstring (the back of the leg)
- Opposite arm move with kicking leg, to 45-90°
- These can be done walking or running

Push Ups – T4

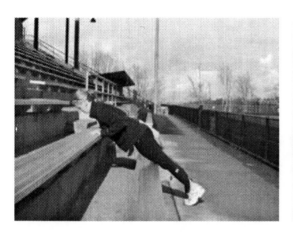 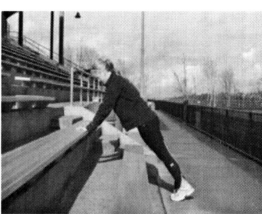

- Keep Body straight
- Hands slightly outside of shoulders
- Hands directly underneath your chest
- Elbows in tight
- Stay on your toes

- Exhale as you push up
- Maintain a straight body
- Keeping your butt down

Side Step Up – T5

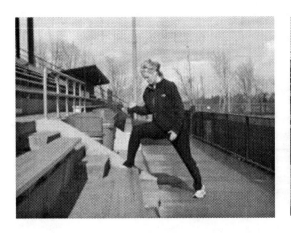 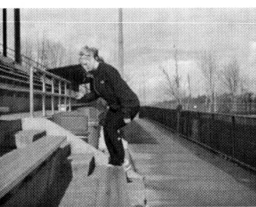

- Keep feet in alignment with knee
- Keep lead foot all the way up on the step
- Keep body turned at a side
- Step up from your heel
- Keep hips back

- Keep hips back
- Do not apply pressure to the helper leg
- You can step up and leave the lead leg up, or you can step down and take the lead leg off and repeat the process
- Focus on something in the ground to help you with your balance
- You should not do this exercise if you knee moves in or out

Sprint Starts – T6

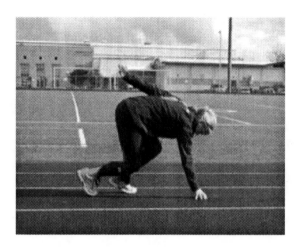

- Keep on toes
- Keep feet about 1 ft apart
- Keep back straight
- Opposite arm goes down to the lead leg
- Keep head down and straight with spine
- This arm supports your body weight that is lurching forward
- Your lead leg is your dominate leg
- (You can figure out your lead leg by pretending you are about to trip and fall and naturally your lead leg will be the leg that steps forward first)

Step Up – T7

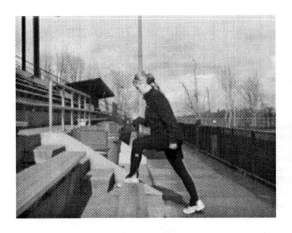 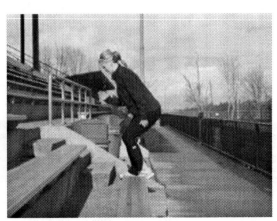

- Keep feet straight
- Keep lead foot all the way up on the step
- Step up from your heel
- Keep hips back

- Keep hips back
- Do not apply pressure to the helper leg
- You can step up and leave the lead leg up, or you can step down and take the lead leg off and repeat the process
- Focus on something in the ground to help you with your balance
- You should not do this exercise if your knee moves in or out

Triceps Dips – T8

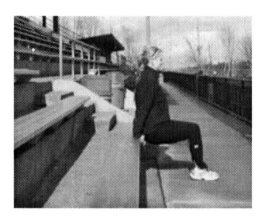 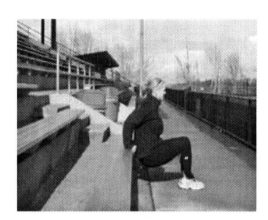

- Keep your back straight and in close to the bench
- Keep elbows in tight
- Keep feet straight
- Keep knees together

- Do not go down past a 60-75° angle
- Squeeze the back of your arms
- Return to original position

Up Up Down Downs – T9

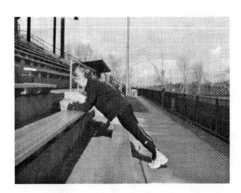

- Keep back straight
- Arms both at 90°
- Elbows in tight
- Keep butt down

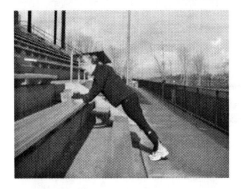

- Come up on 1 hand

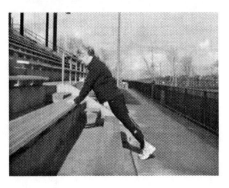

- Then the other...
- Repeat for same arm, then switch

Triceps: Tri

Medball Triceps Extension – Tri1

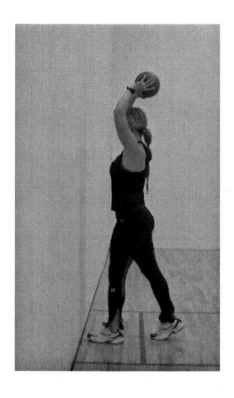 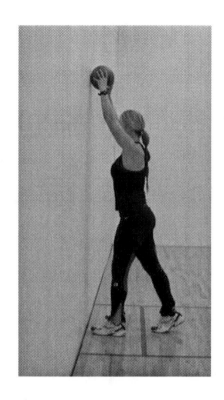

- 1 Leg forward, 1 Leg Back
- Extend your arms Up, holding onto the ball
- Use your Triceps and Core to throw the ball repeatedly against the wall
- Stare straight ahead

- Release the ball fast, catch and repeat

Triceps Extension – Tri2

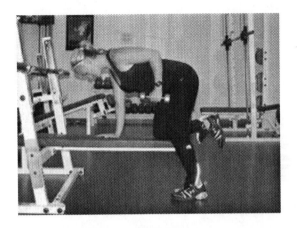 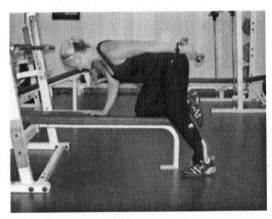

- Keep back straight
- Keep elbow in tight
- Keep arm at 90°
- Keep opposite hand underneath shoulder joint

- Fully extend your arm
- Keep your shoulder down
- Keep spine straight

Triceps Dips - Tri3

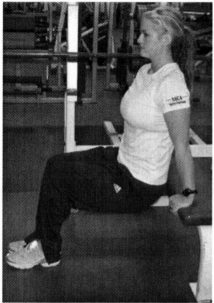

- Keep your back straight and in close to the bench
- Keep elbows in tight
- Keep feet straight
- Keep knees together

- Do not go down past a 60-75° angle
- Squeeze the back of your arms
- Return to original position

Up Up Down Downs - Tri4

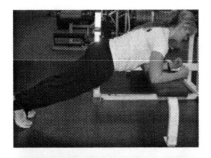

- Keep back straight
- Arms both at 90°
- Elbows in tight

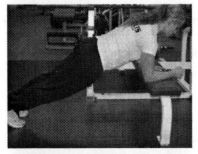

- Come up on one hand...

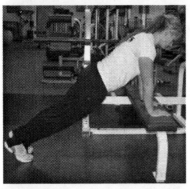

- Then the other...

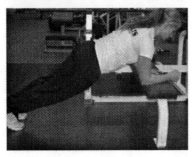

- Come down on the same arm you started with
- Keep your butt down

Afterword

I hope you have enjoyed my book and have learned how you can truly have the best body and personal fitness you've ever had! I have enjoyed writing this book and imploring America to take care of their bodies!

Exercise and good nutrition are a way of life for me and I hope some of that comes across through this book. It was written to be part of the Healthy Lifestyle series created by Trisha Stewart and I recommend that you invest in one of the books from the series that most suits you. The books are as follows:

Healthy Tart

You don't have to be a skinny bitch to be a Healthy Tart! It's the answer to all the 'real women' like you have been hoping to find! Packed with the truth about good nutrition and what actually happens to your body when you eat well (and don't eat so well), you finally have the tools and resources to wade through the size zero/fad diet hype and live your best life now!

Healthy Dude Book

IT'S THE PICK-IT-UP, GET-IT-DONE, LIVING-RIGHT BOOK YOU'VE BEEN WAITING FOR ... The Healthy Dude Book!! Finally ... a one-stop resource to answer your questions about health, nutrition, fitness, disease and more. You take your health seriously, but don't to become an obsessive gym-rat! You're ready to get back in shape, to have the energy to enjoy a long and healthy life - and everything that comes along with it!

Healthy Idol

It's time to 'Get Your Healthy Groove On' with Trisha Stewart's latest and greatest Teen to Twenties' guide to Health, Success and Physical Wellbeing! Talent, drive and ambition are all keys to success in the world of "fame and fortune," but, if you want to GET to the top and STAY on top ... you've got to be a Healthy Idol! From eating to exercise to excess, Healthy Idol guides you to get on track and stay on track as you achieve your dreams. Forget about being a fallen idol - like too many celebrities today. You're a star that deserves to shine for years! This book is the tool you need to do just that.

Healthy Bunch Cookbook   This book is deliberately focusing on vegetarian/vegan foods to support these great lifestyle books but also to encourage those people who eat flesh and dairy to try some great alternatives. Even though Trisha has outlined in her other books very good reasons to avoid eating animal produce she knows some people will continue to do so. Choosing recipes in this book will be greatly contributing to your own health and wellness and that of your family and friends. You will be amazed how many people love to eat this kind of food. Help to spread the word about a great way of eating for optimum health and make this book part of your everyday eating regime.

Checkout www.trishastewart.com for a wealth of health and wellness related topics as well as a complete video workout program designed to complement the workouts in this book.

If you have any comments, questions or observations, please contact me through my website at www.christinmcdowell.com. I will do my best to respond as quickly as I can.

Thanks again for reading my book! I hope I have helped in some way to advance your enthusiasm for working out and ultimately improve your health and fitness!